# Paramedic Care
## Principles & Practice
### Operations

## Workbook
### Fourth Edition

# Paramedic Care
## Principles & Practice
### Operations

## Workbook
### Fourth Edition

*ROBERT S. PORTER*

REVISED BY

**TONY CRYSTAL, SC.D., EMT-P**
EMS Program Coordinator
Richland Community College
Decatur, Illinois

**BRYAN E. BLEDSOE, DO, FACEP, FAAEM, EMT-P**
Professor of Emergency Medicine
Director, Prehospital and Disaster Medicine Fellowship
University of Nevada School of Medicine
Attending Emergency Physician
University Medical Center of Southern Nevada
Medical Director, MedicWest Ambulance
Las Vegas, Nevada

**ROBERT S. PORTER, MA, EMT-P**
Senior Advanced Life Support Educator
Madison County Emergency Medical Services
Canastota, New York

**RICHARD A. CHERRY, MS, NREMT-P**
Director of Training
Northern Onondaga Volunteer Ambulance
Liverpool, New York

**PEARSON**

Boston   Columbus   Indianapolis   New York   San Francisco   Upper Saddle River
Amsterdam   Cape Town   Dubai   London   Madrid   Milan   Munich   Paris   Montréal   Toronto
Delhi   Mexico City   São Paulo   Sydney   Hong Kong   Seoul   Singapore   Taipei   Tokyo

**Publisher:** *Julie Levin Alexander*
**Publisher's Assistant:** *Regina Bruno*
**Editor-in-Chief:** *Marlene McHugh Pratt*
**Senior Managing Editor for Development:** *Lois Berlowitz*
**Editorial Project Manager:** *Triple SSS Press Media Development, Inc.*
**Assistant Editor:** *Jonathan Cheung*
**Director of Marketing:** *David Gesell*
**Marketing Manager:** *Brian Hoehl*
**Marketing Specialist:** *Michael Sirinides*
**Managing Editor for Production:** *Patrick Walsh*
**Production Liaison:** *Faye Gemmellaro*
**Production Editor:** *Muralidharan Krishnamurthy/S4Carlisle Publishing Services*
**Manufacturing Manager:** *Ilene Sanford*
**Cover Design:** *Kathryn Foot*
**Cover Image:** © *corepics/Shutterstock*
**Composition:** *S4Carlisle Publishing Services*
**Cover and Interior Printer/Binder:** *Edwards Brothers Malloy*

# NOTICE ON CARE PROCEDURES

It is the intent of the authors and publisher that this Workbook be used as part of a formal Paramedic program taught by qualified instructors and supervised by a licensed physician. The procedures described in this Workbook are based upon consultation with EMS and medical authorities. The authors and publisher have taken care to make certain that these procedures reflect currently accepted clinical practice; however, they cannot be considered absolute recommendations.

The material in this Workbook contains the most current information available at the time of publication. However, federal, state, and local guidelines concerning clinical practices, including, without limitation, those governing infection control and universal precautions, change rapidly. The reader should note, therefore, that the new regulations may require changes in some procedures.

It is the responsibility of the reader to familiarize himself or herself with the policies and procedures set by federal, state, and local agencies as well as the institution or agency where the reader is employed. The authors and the publisher of this Workbook disclaim any liability, loss, or risk resulting directly or indirectly from the suggested procedures and theory, from any undetected errors, or from the reader's misunderstanding of the text. It is the reader's responsibility to stay informed of any new changes or recommendations made by any federal, state, and local agency as well as by his or her employing institution or agency.

## NOTICE ON CPR AND ECC

The national standards for cardiopulmonary resuscitation (CPR) and emergency cardiovascular care (ECC) are reviewed and revised on a regular basis and may change slightly after this manual is printed. It is important that you know the most current procedures for CPR and ECC, both for the classroom and your patients. The most current information may be obtained from the appropriate credentialing agency.

**Brady**
is an imprint of

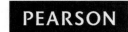

www.bradybooks.com

10 9 8 7 6 5 4 3 2 1
ISBN 10: 0-13-211133-0
ISBN 13: 978-0-13-211133-1

# *Dedication*

*This workbook is dedicated to the important people in your life: your wife/husband, mother, father, sister, brother . . . and friends who support you and the time and passion you devote to Emergency Medical Service.*
*Without them, this endeavor would be lonely and much less rewarding.*

–ROBERT S. PORTER

# CONTENTS

# INTRODUCTION

Welcome to the self-instructional Workbook for *Paramedic Care: Principles & Practice*. This Workbook is designed to help guide you through an educational program for initial or refresher training that follows the guidelines of the 2009 *National EMS Education Standards*. The Workbook is designed to be used either in conjunction with your instructor or as a self-study guide you use on your own.

This Workbook features many different ways to help you learn the material necessary to become a paramedic, as described next.

# Features

## Review of Chapter Objectives

Each chapter of *Paramedic Care: Principles & Practice* begins with objectives that identify the important information and principles addressed in the chapter reading. To help you identify and learn this material, each Workbook chapter reviews the important content elements addressed by these objectives as presented in the text.

## Case Study Review

Each chapter of *Paramedic Care: Principles & Practice* includes a case study, introducing and highlighting important principles presented in the chapter. The Workbook reviews these case studies and points out much of the essential information and many of the applied principles they describe.

## Content Self-Evaluation

Each chapter of *Paramedic Care: Principles & Practice* presents an extensive narrative explanation of the principles of paramedic practice. The Workbook chapter (or chapter section) contains between 10 and 50 multiple-choice questions to test your reading comprehension of the textbook material and to give you experience taking typical emergency medical service examinations.

## Special Projects

The Workbook contains several projects that are special learning experiences designed to help you remember the information and principles necessary to perform as a paramedic. Special projects include contacting local agencies and services, Internet research, and a variety of other exercises.

## Content Review

The Workbook provides a comprehensive review of the material presented in this volume of *Paramedic Care: Principles & Practice*. After the last text chapter has been covered, the Workbook presents an extensive content self-evaluation component that helps you recall and build upon the knowledge you have gained by reading the text, attending class, and completing the earlier Workbook chapters.

# HOW TO USE THIS SELF-INSTRUCTIONAL WORKBOOK

The self-instructional Workbook accompanying *Paramedic Care: Principles & Practice* may be used as directed by your instructor or independently by you during your course of instruction. The following recommendations are intended to guide you in using the Workbook independently.

- Examine your course schedule and identify the appropriate text chapter or other assigned reading.

- Read the assigned chapter in *Paramedic Care: Principles & Practice* carefully. Do this in a relaxed environment, free of distractions, and give yourself adequate time to read and digest the material. The information presented in *Paramedic Care: Principles & Practice* is often technically complex and demanding, but it is very important that you comprehend it. Be sure that you read the chapter carefully enough to understand and remember what you have read.

- Carefully read the Review of Chapter Objectives at the beginning of each Workbook chapter (or section). This material includes both the objectives listed in *Paramedic Care: Principles & Practice* and narrative descriptions of their content. If you do not understand or remember what is discussed from your reading, refer to the referenced pages and reread them carefully. If you still do not feel comfortable with your understanding of any objective, consider asking your instructor about it.

- Reread the case study in *Paramedic Care: Principles & Practice*, and then read the Case Study Review in the Workbook. Note the important points regarding assessment and care that the Case Study Review highlights and be sure that you understand and agree with the analysis of the call. If you have any questions or concerns, ask your instructor to clarify the information.

- Take the Content Self-Evaluation at the end of each Workbook chapter (or section), answering each question carefully. Do this in a quiet environment, free from distractions, and allow yourself adequate time to complete the exercise. Correct your self-evaluation by consulting the answers at the back of the Workbook, and determine the percentage you have answered correctly (the number you got right divided by the total number of questions). If you have answered most of the questions correctly (85 to 90 percent), review those that you missed by rereading the material on the pages listed in the answer key and be sure you understand which answer is correct and why. If you have more than a few questions wrong (less than 85 percent correct), look for incorrect answers that are grouped together. This suggests that you did not understand a particular topic in the reading. Reread the text dealing with that topic carefully, and then retest yourself on the questions you got wrong. If incorrect answers are spread throughout the chapter content, reread the chapter and retake the Content Self-Evaluation to ensure that you understand the material. If you don't understand why your answer to a question is incorrect after reviewing the text, consult with your instructor.

- In a similar fashion, complete the exercises in the Special Projects section of the Workbook chapters (or sections). These exercises are specifically designed to help you learn and remember the essential principles and information presented in *Paramedic Care: Principles & Practice*.

- When you have completed this volume of *Paramedic Care: Principles & Practice* and its accompanying Workbook, prepare for a course test by reviewing both the text in its entirety and your class notes. Then take the Content Review examination in the Workbook. Again, review your score and any questions you have answered incorrectly by referring to the text and rereading the page or pages where the material is presented. If you note groupings of wrong answers, review the entire range of pages or the full chapter they represent.

*If, during your completion of the Workbook exercises, you have any questions that either the textbook or Workbook doesn't answer, write them down and ask your instructor about them. Prehospital emergency medicine is a complex and complicated subject, and answers are not always black and white. It is also common for different EMS systems to use differing methods of care. The questions you bring up in class, and your instructor's answers to them, will help you expand and complete your knowledge of prehospital emergency medical care.*

# GUIDELINES TO BETTER TEST-TAKING

The knowledge you will gain from reading the textbook, completing the exercises in the Workbook, listening in your paramedic class, and participating in your clinical and field experience will prepare you to care for patients who are seriously ill or injured. However, before you can practice these skills, you will have to pass several classroom written exams and your state's certification exam. Your performance on these exams will depend not only on your knowledge but also on your ability to answer test questions correctly. The following guidelines are designed to help your performance on tests and to better demonstrate your knowledge of pre-hospital emergency care.

## 1. Relax and be calm during the test.

A test is designed to measure what you have learned and to tell you and your instructor how well you are doing. An exam is not designed to intimidate or punish you. Consider it a challenge, and just try to do your best. Get plenty of sleep before the examination. Avoid coffee or other stimulants for a few hours before the exam, and be prepared.

Reread the text chapters, review the objectives in the Workbook, and review your class notes. It might be helpful to work with one or two other students and ask each other questions. This type of practice helps everyone better understand the knowledge presented in your course of study.

## 2. Read the questions carefully.

Read each word of the question and all the answers slowly. Words such as "except" or "not" may change the entire meaning of the question. If you miss such words, you may answer the question incorrectly even though you know the right answer.

*Example:*

The art and science of emergency medical services involves all of the following EXCEPT

    **A.** sincerity and compassion.

    **B.** respect for human dignity.

    **C.** placing patient care before personal safety.

    **D.** delivery of sophisticated emergency medical care.

    **E.** none of the above.

The correct answer is C, unless you miss the "EXCEPT."

## 3. Read each answer carefully.

Read each and every answer carefully. Although the first answer may be absolutely correct, so may the rest, and thus the best answer might be "all of the above."

*Example:*

Indirect medical direction is considered to be

    **A.** treatment protocols.

    **B.** training and education.

    **C.** quality assurance.

    **D.** chart review.

    **E.** all of the above.

Although answers A, B, C, and D are each correct, the best and only acceptable answer is "all of the above," E.

## 4. Delay answering questions you don't understand and look for clues.

When a question seems confusing or you don't know the answer, note it on your answer sheet and come back to it later. This will ensure that you have time to complete the test. You will also find that other questions in the test may give you hints to answer the one you've skipped over. It will also prevent you from being frustrated with an early question and letting it affect your performance.

*Example:*

Upon successful completion of a course of training as an EMT-P, most states will

    **A.**   certify you. (correct)
    **B.**   license you.
    **C.**   register you.
    **D.**   recognize you as a paramedic.
    **E.**   issue you a permit.

Another question, later in the exam, may suggest the right answer:

The action of one state in recognizing the certification of another is called:

    **A.**   reciprocity. (correct)
    **B.**   national registration.
    **C.**   licensure.
    **D.**   registration.
    **E.**   extended practice.

## 5. Answer all questions.

Even if you do not know the right answer, do not leave a question blank. A blank question is always wrong, whereas a guess might be correct. If you can eliminate some of the answers as wrong, do so. It will increase the chances of a correct guess.

A multiple-choice question with five answers gives a 20 percent chance of a correct guess. If you can eliminate one or more incorrect answers, you increase your odds of a correct guess to 25 percent, 33 percent, and so on. An unanswered question has a 0 percent chance of being correct.

Just before turning in your answer sheet, check to be sure that you have not left any items blank.

*Example:*

When a paramedic is called by the patient (through the dispatcher) to the scene of a medical emergency, the medical direction physician has established a physician/patient relationship.

    **A.**   True
    **B.**   False

A true/false question gives you a 50 percent chance of a correct guess.

The hospital health professional(s) responsible for sorting patients as they arrive at the emergency department is (are) usually the

    **A.**   emergency physician.
    **B.**   ward clerk.
    **C.**   emergency nurse.
    **D.**   trauma surgeon.
    **E.**   both A and C (correct).

# Paramedic Care
## Principles & Practice
### Operations

## Workbook

**Fourth Edition**

# 1

# Ground Ambulance Operations

## Review of Chapter Objectives

### After reading this chapter, you should be able to:

1. **Define key terms introduced in this chapter.** pp. 1–2

   Knowing and being able to apply the key terms in each chapter is critical to understanding chapter concepts. Write the list of key terms. Then write the definition of each one in your own words. Check your understanding by confirming the definitions in the text glossary. Correct any misunderstandings. Create a study aid by writing each key term on the front of an index card and the definition on the back. Use the cards to quiz yourself, or to have someone quiz you.

2. **Describe the roles of standards, trends, and administrative rules and regulations on the design of ambulances and the equipment they carry.** p. 2

   Various standards, as well as administrative rules and regulations, influence the design of ambulances and the medical equipment carried on each unit. Similar guidelines determine staffing levels and deployment of EMS agencies. Because the oversight for EMS usually falls to state governments, many of the requirements for ambulance service are written in state statutes or regulations. These regulations, known as the "state EMS code," might then handle such matters as the essential equipment to be carried on every ambulance. State standards usually set minimum standards, rather than a gold standard, for operation. In other words, they establish the lowest level at which units will be allowed to operate. When local and/or regional EMS systems get involved in regulation, their lists tend to be much more detailed and often approach a gold standard, which is the goal when ample resources are provided.

3. **Identify the types of ambulance design according to the General Services Administration federal specifications for ambulances.** pp. 2–3

   The U.S. General Services Administration's Automotive Commodity Center issues the federal regulations that specify ambulance design and manufacturing requirements. These specifications, known as the DOT KKK 1822F specs, attempt to influence safety standards as well as standardize the look of ambulances.

   The specs describe the following three basic ambulance designs: Type I (conventional truck cab-chassis with a modular ambulance body), Type II (standard van, forward control integral cab-body ambulance), and Type III (specialty van, forward control integral cab-body ambulance). In addition to these three designs, there is also a medium-duty ambulance rescue vehicle that is designed to handle heavier loads and has a gross weight of approximately 24,000 pounds. These are designed as a Type I-AD (additional duty) or Type II-AD depending upon their basic structure.

The federal specifications not only provide standards for the purchase of ambulances used by the federal government, but they also provide guidelines for the states to follow. In such cases, the federal specifications become the state standard for ambulance services to follow when purchasing vehicles. Some states have chosen to develop their own standards. Often these states use the federal specifications as the basis or starting point for their own regulations. A few states use neither federal nor state specifications. Instead, the decisions for ambulance purchases are determined on a local or regional basis.

In addition to the U.S. Department of Transportation (DOT), other federal agencies and national organizations influence standards. Air ambulance standards, for example, are usually designed with input from representatives of the Air and Surface Transport Nurses Association (ASTNA), the International Association of Flight and Critical Care Paramedics (IAFCCP), and the Association of Air Medical Services (AAMS). The Federal Communications Commission (FCC) specifies the radio bands and types of equipment that may be used in ambulances.

**4. Describe the roles of the Commission on Accreditation for Ambulance Services and the American College of Surgeons Committee on Trauma with respect to ambulance equipment and supplies.** p. 4

At the national level, the Commission on Accreditation of Ambulance Services (CAAS) provides a voluntary "gold standard" for the EMS community to follow. CAAS requires that on-board medical equipment and supplies comply with state and local guidelines. In the absence of these guidelines, CAAS requires services to develop guidelines that meet or exceed those established by the American College of Surgeons (ACS). The ACS Committee of Trauma issued its first list of "essential equipment" to be carried on ambulances in 1970 and revised the list in 1994. Of note is that as long ago as 1970 the list included the ALS equipment, emergency drugs, and fluids commonly used on ALS calls today.

**5. Describe the role and responsibilities of the paramedic in checking the ambulance at the beginning of each shift.** pp. 4–5

On each shift, an essential part of a paramedic's duties includes completion of the ambulance equipment and supply checklist. Aside from reminding the personnel exactly where all equipment and supplies are stored on the ambulance, the shift checklist helps ensure that all equipment and supplies will be available and in working order when needed for patient care. The checklist also makes the work environment safer by ensuring mechanical maintenance and the availability of personal protective equipment (PPE).

Routine detailed shift checks of the ambulance can minimize the issues associated with risk management. Medications carried on the paramedic unit expire; therefore, expiration dates should be checked each shift, and the older, unexpired drugs marked appropriately so that they will be used first. In services that use scheduled medications such as narcotics, the paramedics should sign for these medications at the beginning and at the end of each shift.

The vehicle itself should be regularly checked so that it is always in safe working order. If the ambulance or any equipment needs repair, it is your responsibility to report the failure to your supervisor in a manner prescribed by the standard operating procedures (SOPs) for your service.

To meet Occupational Safety and Health Administration (OSHA) requirements, you must also make sure that the ambulance has been properly disinfected after the transport of any patients with potentially communicable diseases. If there is no specific SOP in your agency, you should document cleaning and disinfecting on the shift checklist.

Finally, you should do all scheduled tests, maintenance, and calibrations on specific medical equipment.

**6. Identify components of typical ambulance checklists.** pp. 4–5

Components of a typical vehicle/equipment checklist include the following:

- Patient infection control, comfort, and protection supplies
- Initial and focused assessment equipment

©2013 Pearson Education, Inc.
*Paramedic Care: Principles & Practice, Vol. 7, 4th Ed.*

- Equipment for the transfer of the patient
- Equipment for airway maintenance, ventilation, and resuscitation
- Oxygen therapy and suction equipment
- Equipment for assisting with cardiac resuscitation
- Supplies and equipment for immobilization of suspected bone injuries
- Supplies for wound care and treatment of shock
- Supplies for childbirth
- Supplies, equipment, and medications for the treatment of acute poisoning, snakebite, chemical burns, and diabetic emergencies
- ALS equipment, medications, and supplies
- Safety and miscellaneous equipment
- Information on the operation and inspection of the ambulance itself

Components of regularly scheduled tests, maintenance, and calibrations on specific medical equipment include:

- Automated external defibrillator (AED)
- Glucometer
- Cardiac monitor, defibrillator, and pacer
- Capnograph
- Oxygen systems
- Automated transport ventilator (ATV)
- Pulse oximeter
- Suction units
- Laryngoscope blades
- Lighted stylets
- Penlights
- Any other battery-operated equipment

7. **Describe considerations in ambulance deployment and staffing configurations.**
pp. 5–6

Deployment is based on a number of factors: location of the facilities to house ambulances, location of hospitals, anticipated volume of calls, and the specific geographic and traffic considerations of your area. Most services must develop deployment strategies based on current station locations.

The ideal deployment decisions must take into account two sets of data: past community responses and projected demographic changes. The highest volume of calls, or peak load, should be described both in terms of the day of the week and the time of day. In communities that do not have multiple strategically located stations, services often deploy ambulances to wait for calls at specific high-volume locations. Such stationing locations are known as primary areas of responsibility (PARs). These ambulances may be relocated throughout the day as the population moves—to work or to school—and as other ambulances in the community respond to calls. The PAR size depends on the number of ambulances available and the expected call volume.

In determining deployment strategies, traffic congestion must be taken into account, as well as special situations such as a ground-level railroad. One deployment strategy that has become popular in recent years is known as system status management (SSM). SSM is a computerized personnel and ambulance deployment system designed to meet service demands with fewer resources and to ensure appropriate response times and vehicle locations.

The EMS response time can make the difference between life and death for the citizens of a community—especially in the setting of cardiac arrest. However, recent research has shown that only response times of less than 4 minutes are associated with improved outcomes. Several studies have shown that an 8-minute response time, a de facto industry standard, is not uniformly associated with better patient outcomes overall. In most areas, a routine response time of 4 minutes is either impossible or cost-prohibitive. Thus, appropriate response times must be determined by each community and its available resources.

To meet reliability standards, many communities use a tiered response system in which public safety workers trained as first responders carry an AED to a patient's side. The first tier of response, which helps ensure arrival within the 4-minute window, is then backed up by a second tier that brings an ALS unit to the patient within 8 minutes. Some communities add a third tier of response by separating their paramedics from their ambulances. No one system works best for all communities. The system that is ideal for your specific area will depend on such considerations as available personnel, available training, and many other factors.

Ambulance staffing should take into account the peak load of the system. Some services vary shift times to ensure ample coverage for the busiest days of the week and the busiest times of the day. Services should also take into account the need for reserve capacity—the ability to muster additional crews when all ambulances are on call or when a system's resources are taxed by a multiple-casualty incident. Some services fulfill this need by asking off-duty personnel to carry pagers or to volunteer for backup. Whatever plan is adopted, each system must consider how it will deal with establishing a reserve of paramedics. Finally, each service needs to determine standards for ambulance operators (drivers) and for driving the vehicle itself. As a rule, these standards are usually spelled out at the local service level.

8. **Discuss the significance of ambulance collisions.** pp. 6–7

Patients, family members, motorists, and EMS providers are injured—sometimes fatally—in ambulance collisions. In addition to personal injuries, ambulance collisions exact a high toll: vehicle repair or replacement, lawsuits, downtime from work, increased insurance premiums, and damage to your agency's reputation in the community.

There has been a marked increase in the frequency of ground ambulance accidents over the past decade. The exact cause is unclear, although several theories have been proposed. First, modern automobiles are better sealed and more soundproof than cars of even a decade ago. This can make it difficult for persons to hear an approaching ambulance. In addition, ambulances have increased in size and weight. The performance characteristic of modern ambulances is quite different from that of older models. Modern ambulances tend to be on a truck chassis and have characteristics more consistent with a large truck than a car. They accelerate poorly, are less responsive, and have a much greater braking distance. Also, the center of gravity is quite different from that of automobiles.

No national database has been set up to provide statistics on ambulance collisions in all 50 states. As a result, it is difficult to establish any form of "acceptable" ambulance collision rate per number of calls or miles driven. Furthermore, few scientific studies have been published that attempt to prove what, if any, strategies effectively reduce ambulance collisions.

An analysis of 22 years of reportable collisions—collisions involving more than $1,000 in vehicle damage or a personal injury—in New York State provides a profile of the typical ambulance collision. Inclement weather accounted for a relatively small number of the accidents. About 18 percent occurred on rainy days, 16 percent on cloudy days, and 6 percent on days with snow, sleet, hail, or freezing rain. The majority of collisions (55 percent) took place on clear days. Of all the collisions, some 67 percent took place during daylight hours.

Although head-on collisions can be very serious, they accounted for only 1 percent of the accidents. The largest number of collisions (41 percent) occurred when the ambulance struck another vehicle laterally or at a right angle or was struck itself. Approximately 21 percent of the collisions resulted from side swiping or overtaking another vehicle. Another 12 percent occurred while making a right or left turn.

Probably the most important observation from the data is that nearly three-quarters (72 percent) of all collisions took place at intersections. Most safety-minded ambulance operators agree that the days of "blowing through" an intersection at high speeds with lights blaring and siren blasting have come and gone. Yet nearly half of all accidents took place at locations with a traffic control device. Another third took place at locations with no traffic device or sign.

Based on the statistics from New York, the profile of a typical ambulance collision might read as follows: A lateral collision that takes place on a dry road during daylight hours on a clear day in an intersection with a traffic light.

©2013 Pearson Education, Inc.
*Paramedic Care: Principles & Practice, Vol. 7, 4th Ed.*

9. **Identify strategies for reducing the risk of ambulance collisions and associated deaths and injuries.** p. 7

In developing programs to reduce ambulance collisions in your community, consider implementing the following actions or standards:

- Routine use of driver qualification checklists and driver's license checks, either through the local police or the Department of Motor Vehicles
- Demonstrated driver understanding of preventive mechanical maintenance, including a vehicle operator checklist and a procedure for reporting any problems found during the check or while driving the vehicle
- Provision of adequate hands-on driver training, using experienced and qualified field officers.
- Implementation of a slow-speed course to ensure that operators know how to use mirrors, back up, park, and handle ambulance-sized vehicles, including accurate estimation of braking distance and turn radius
- Training that ensures operators know how to react to emergency situations such as the loss of brakes, loss of power steering, a stuck accelerator, a blown-out tire, or a vehicle breakdown
- Demonstrated driver knowledge of both the primary and backup routes to all hospitals in your service response area
- Demonstrated driver understanding of the rules, regulations, and laws that your Department of Motor Vehicles has established for drivers in general and for ambulance operators in particular

10. **Implement safety measures related to driving, parking, and loading the ambulance.** pp. 8–11

Each EMS agency should have SOPs pertaining to the operation of its vehicles. At a minimum, SOPs should spell out the following:

- Procedure for qualifying as an ambulance operator
- Procedure for handling and reporting an ambulance collision
- Process for investigating and reviewing each collision
- Process for implementing quality assurance in the aftermath of a collision
- Method for using a spotter when backing up a vehicle
- Use of seat belts in the ambulance, and the procedure for transporting a child passenger under 40 pounds
- Guidelines on what constitutes an emergency response and the exemptions that may be taken under state laws
- Guidelines on prudent speed; proper travel in, and the circumstances for using, oncoming lanes; and safe negotiation of intersections
- Circumstances and procedures for use of escorts
- A zero-tolerance policy for driving the vehicle under the influence of alcohol or any drugs

The motor vehicle laws enacted by most states are based on a model law. As might be expected, state laws pertaining to ambulance operation tend to be similar. One similarity centers on the legal concept of due regard. Essentially, due regard exempts ambulance drivers from certain laws, but at the same time holds them to a higher standard.

As a general rule, do not rely solely on lights and siren to alert other motorists of your approach. The siren is the most commonly used—and abused—audible warning device. Some states and services have specific laws and/or SOPs that address the use of sirens. Consider these useful guidelines: use the siren sparingly and only when you must; never assume that all motorists will hear your siren; assume that some motorists will hear your siren, but choose to ignore it; be prepared for panic and erratic maneuvers when drivers do hear your siren; and never use the siren to scare someone.

Most EMS agencies no longer suggest the use of a police escort for ambulances, except in circumstances in which the ambulance is providing service to an unfamiliar district and needs to be taken to the patient and/or the hospital. There are several reasons for this, including: different braking distances, different acceleration speeds, and other motorists are not likely to realize that the two emergency vehicles are traveling together.

In multiple-vehicle responses, the dangers are the same as for an escort. In addition, another danger occurs when two emergency vehicles approach an intersection at the same time. Besides totally confusing motorists and pedestrians, the potential for an intersection collision increases dramatically. Motorists often fail to yield the right of way to the first emergency vehicle, the second emergency vehicle, or, in some instances, both vehicles. As a general rule, always negotiate an intersection assuming that you may meet another emergency vehicle.

Recall that New York statistics reveal that 72 percent of all ambulance collisions occur in intersections. Clearly the intersection is a very unsafe, if not deadly, place to be. Exercise extreme caution whenever you approach one of these hazards. Keep in mind the braking distance of your ambulance, the effectiveness of lights and siren, the rules of the road, the SOPs of your service, the acceleration needed to get through the intersection safely, and more. Helpful tips for negotiating an intersection include the following:

- Stop at all red lights and stop signs and then proceed with caution.
- Always proceed through an intersection slowly.
- Make eye contact with other motorists to ensure they understand your intentions.
- If you are using any of the exemptions offered to you as an emergency vehicle, such as passing through a red light or a stop sign, make sure you warn motorists by appropriately flashing your lights and sounding the siren.
- Remember that lights and siren only "ask" the public to yield the right of way.
- Always go around cars stopped at the intersection on their left (driver's) side.
- Know how long it takes for your ambulance to cross an intersection.
- Watch pedestrians at an intersection carefully.
- Remember that there is no such thing as a rolling stop in an ambulance weighing more than 10,000 pounds or a medium-duty vehicle weighing some 24,000 pounds. These vehicles will not stop on a dime.

Whenever you arrive first at the site of a motor vehicle collision, take steps to size up the scene for potential hazards to you, your crew, and the patients. Consider establishing a danger zone and parking at least 100 feet from the wreckage upwind and uphill (if possible) to avoid fire or any escaping hazardous liquids or fumes. If there is no fire or escaping liquids or fumes, park at least 50 feet from the wreckage. If possible, assign a member of the crew to handle traffic until the police arrive to take control of the task. If your ambulance is the first emergency vehicle on the scene, make sure you park in front of the wreckage so your warning lights can alert approaching motorists. If the scene has already been secured, park beyond the wreckage to prevent your ambulance from being exposed to traffic.

Always be aware of potential traffic hazards at the scene of a call. Many EMS providers have been seriously injured—and some even killed—after being struck by passing motorists. As much as possible, try not to expose either your crew or your patient to traffic. Keep in mind that the rear ambulance doors often obstruct the warning lights when they are opened to load the patient.

©2013 Pearson Education, Inc.
*Paramedic Care: Principles & Practice, Vol. 7, 4th Ed.*

# Case Study Review

*Reread the case study on page 2 in* Paramedic Care: Operations; *then, read the following discussion.*

   *This case study draws attention to the importance of well-stocked ambulances to provide effective patient care.*

As indicated in the closing paragraph of the case study, some services do not value the importance of having the right equipment and supplies available at all times for every patient. Eventually that attitude catches up with them and someone gets hurt.

   Most quality services are very strict about restocking ambulances. A rig check should be the first order of business upon arrival for each shift. This helps to ensure that the last crew did its job correctly. It is also a good practice to restock after each call as well as to refuel the vehicle. In this way, you will not run short of any essential item—and you will experience a smooth and uneventful run, like the dedicated service described in the case study.

# Content Self-Evaluation

## MULTIPLE CHOICE

_____   1. What type of ambulance standards are usually set by states?
   A.  Minimum standards
   B.  Maximum standards
   C.  Gold standards
   D.  Essential-equipment standards
   E.  DOT KKK standards

_____   2. A conventional truck cab-chassis with a modular ambulance body is a _____ ambulance design.
   A.  Type I
   B.  Type II
   C.  Type III
   D.  medium-duty
   E.  heavy-duty

_____   3. A specialty van with a forward control integral cab-body is a _____ ambulance design.
   A.  Type I
   B.  Type II
   C.  Type III
   D.  medium-duty
   E.  heavy-duty

_____   4. Which of the following agencies or organizations influence(s) ambulance standards?
   A.  Department of Transportation (DOT)
   B.  Air and Surface Transport Nurses Association (ASTNA)
   C.  International Association of Flight and Critical Care Paramedics (IAFCCP)
   D.  Federal Communications Commission (FCC)
   E.  All of the above

5. The agency that has helped ensure equipment lists calling for disinfecting agents, sharps containers, and other protective items on-board ambulances is
   A. NIOSH.
   B. NFPA.
   C. OSHA.
   D. CDC.
   E. NFPA.

6. The agency that provides a "gold standard" for the EMS community to follow, including a list of "essential equipment" to be carried on ambulances is
   A. ACS.
   B. CAAS.
   C. NFPA.
   D. NIOSH.
   E. OSHA.

7. The expiration dates on medications carried on the paramedic unit should be checked
   A. once a day.
   B. once a week.
   C. at the start of every shift.
   D. at the start of every month.
   E. every other day.

8. An EMS agency uses deployment based on all of the following factors, EXCEPT
   A. anticipated call volume.
   B. local geographic and traffic conditions.
   C. location of hospitals.
   D. projected ethnic makeup of the population.
   E. location of facilities to house ambulances.

9. A deployment strategy that uses a computerized personnel and ambulance deployment system is known as
   A. a peak load system.
   B. a primary area of responsibility.
   C. system status management.
   D. primary deploy management.
   E. none of the above.

10. A system that allows multiple vehicles to arrive at an EMS call at different times is called a
    A. multiple response system.
    B. tiered response system.
    C. primary response system.
    D. reserve capacity system.
    E. peak load system.

11. Almost all communities in the United States require two paramedics aboard an ALS unit.
    A. True
    B. False

12. According to one study, the majority of ambulance collisions occur
    A. in patients' driveways.
    B. at intersections.
    C. when backing into ambulance bays.
    D. at night.
    E. during inclement weather.

13. A legal term found in the motor vehicle laws of most states that sets up a higher standard for the operators of emergency vehicles is called
    A. *res ispa loquitur.*
    B. exempt rights.
    C. emergency power.
    D. due regard.
    E. special status.

©2013 Pearson Education, Inc.
*Paramedic Care: Principles & Practice, Vol. 7, 4th Ed.*

14. State laws typically exempt ambulance drivers who are operating in an emergency from all of the following traffic situations, EXCEPT
    A. posted speed limits.
    B. crossing railroad tracks with the gates down.
    C. posted directions of travel.
    D. parking regulations.
    E. requirements to wait for red lights.

15. Nowhere in the motor vehicle laws are drivers other than emergency vehicle operators held accountable for the safety of all other motorists.
    A. True
    B. False

16. Which of the following is NOT true about the use of lights and sirens?
    A. Motorists are less inclined to yield to an ambulance when the siren is sounded continuously.
    B. Many motorists feel that the right-of-way privileges given to ambulances are abused when sirens are sounded.
    C. Inexperienced motorists tend to decrease their driving speed by 10 to 15 miles per hour when a siren is sounded.
    D. The continuous sound of a siren can possibly worsen the condition of patients by increasing their anxiety.
    E. Ambulance drivers may develop anxiety from using sirens on long runs.

17. Why do most EMS agencies no longer suggest the use of a police escort for ambulances?
    A. Ambulances and police cars have different braking distances.
    B. Motorists are often confused by escorts going through intersections.
    C. Motorists often will not see the second vehicle and pull out in front of it.
    D. Ambulance drivers may have trouble keeping up with police cars.
    E. All of the above.

18. When your ambulance is the first to arrive at the scene of a motor vehicle collision, you should park
    A. behind the wreckage.
    B. in front of the wreckage.
    C. in a staging area.
    D. next to the wreckage on the side.
    E. across the road from the wreckage.

19. Always go around cars stopped at an intersection on their right (passenger's) side.
    A. True
    B. False

20. When negotiating an intersection, avoid eye contact with motorists to better focus on your driving.
    A. True
    B. False

21. Use of lights and sirens requires the public to yield the right of way.
    A. True
    B. False

# MATCHING

*Write the letter of the term in the space provided next to the appropriate description.*

A. peak load

B. primary area of responsibility

C. tiered response system

D. deployment

E. demographic

F. gold standard

G. spotter

H. reportable collisions

I. minimum standard

J. reserve capacity

_____ 22. Strategy used by an EMS agency to maneuver its ambulances and crews in an effort to reduce response times

_____ 23. Ultimate standard of excellence

_____ 24. Lowest or least allowable standards

_____ 25. The highest volume of calls at a given time

_____ 26. Pertaining to population makeup or changes

_____ 27. Stationing of ambulances at specific high-volume locations

_____ 28. Allows multiple vehicles to arrive at an EMS call at different times, often providing different levels of care or transport

_____ 29. The ability of an EMS agency to respond to calls beyond those handled by the on-duty crews

_____ 30. Collisions that involve over $1,000 in damage or a personal injury

_____ 31. The person behind the left rear side of the ambulance who assists the operator in backing up the vehicle

©2013 Pearson Education, Inc.
*Paramedic Care: Principles & Practice, Vol. 7, 4th Ed.*

# Special Project

*The motor vehicle laws differ slightly from state to state. Ask your chief or EMS director for a copy of the laws in your state and review them very closely. List below the exemptions that you may take when responding to an emergency in your ambulance:*

_____

_____

_____

_____

_____

_____

_____

*Now review the standard operating procedures for negotiating an intersection. Write the key elements of the policy below:*

_____

_____

_____

_____

_____

_____

_____

# Air Medical Operations

## Review of Chapter Objectives

### After reading this chapter, you should be able to:

1. **Define key terms introduced in this chapter.**      p. 14

   Knowing and being able to apply the key terms in each chapter is critical to understanding chapter concepts. Write the list of key terms. Then write the definition of each one in your own words. Check your understanding by confirming the definitions in the text glossary. Correct any misunderstandings. Create a study aid by writing each key term on the front of an index card and the definition on the back. Use the cards to quiz yourself, or to have someone quiz you.

2. **Describe the roles and uses that helicopters and fixed-wing aircraft can play in the care and transport of ill or injured patients.**      pp. 15–16

   The use of aircraft for emergency patient transport has become a critical component of modern EMS practice. Both helicopters and airplanes (fixed wing) have proved to be a vital asset in the emergent transport of the ill or injured patient in the following areas.

   **Scene Responses.** The first major use of aircraft, specifically helicopters, was for flying directly to an incident scene and then transporting the patient to a definitive care facility. Scene responses may be primary (air medical crew is first on the scene) or secondary (summoned by ground personnel).

   **Interfacility Transport.** One of the most rapidly expanding areas of air medical transport is the emergent transfer of patients between health care facilities. In the rural setting, patients often require a level of specialty care that is unavailable locally. When dealing with critically ill patients, significant prehospital time can be minimized through air transport. The type of aircraft used is based upon the distance to be traveled and the patient's condition. Generally speaking, helicopters are limited to distances less than 150 to 200 miles.

   **Specialty Care.** Air medical transport can bring specialty teams to community hospitals for care of selected patients. The most common example is that of neonatal transport. Neonates, especially preterm infants, can require sophisticated specialized care. In some systems, a neonatal team is transported to the community hospital, where initial stabilization is completed. Following that, transport may or may not be by aircraft. In some systems, the neonatal team is transported to the community hospital by helicopter, and return to the tertiary care facility is often by ground ambulance.

   **Organ Procurement.** The transplantation of human organs has evolved significantly over the past two decades. The procurement of human organs is a time-sensitive endeavor. Because of this, organ procurement teams often use aircraft to respond to the site of the donor and subsequently transport the organs back to the transport center.

**Search and Rescue.** The use of aircraft for search and rescue has been a part of aviation virtually since its inception. Medical aircraft, including both fixed-wing aircraft and helicopters, are sometimes used in search-and-rescue operations. Although this can be system dependent, it is not an uncommon practice. Medical helicopter pilots and crews are often intimately familiar with local geography and can provide much-needed assistance in search-and-rescue operations. The addition of technology such as high-intensity spotlights, forward looking infra-red (FLIR), and night vision goggles (NVG) makes aircraft a valuable asset in these situations.

**Disaster Assistance.** Disaster situations often impact or destroy the infrastructure of the community and region affected. In many instances, ingress and egress are restricted because of the destruction of roads. This is commonly seen following both earthquakes and hurricanes. However, it is also seen in tornadoes and similar events. Aircraft, particularly helicopters, can provide access to disaster regions not accessible by ground ambulances.

3. **Describe the evolution of air medical transport over time, including key events that led to the development of air medical transport as it exists today.** **p. 17**

The first recorded use of an airplane to evacuate wounded casualties was during World War I by a French aircraft in Serbia. Later in that same war, the British used aircraft to evacuate casualties in the Turkish theater. Subsequently, a fully organized air ambulance operation was used by both the French and British during the African and Middle Eastern colonial wars of the 1920s. During Germany's involvement in the Spanish Civil War, casualties from its "Condor Legion" expeditionary force were evacuated by Junkers Ju-52 trimotors back to Germany for care.

The first successful operational helicopter was the Sikorsky YR-4, built in the United States in 1942. These were then deployed in an experiment to Burma by the U.S. Army in 1944–1945. Initially they were intended to be used in a search-and-rescue function for downed aircrew, but on January 26, 1945, the first documented medical evacuation by helicopter took place in the jungles of Burma that otherwise would have taken 10 days on foot to accomplish.

By the time the United States entered the Korean War in 1950, helicopter usage had become more common both as an aerial observation platform and for the medical evacuation of infantry casualties. In Korea, patients were evacuated from the battlefield to Mobile Army Surgical Hospital (MASH) units and battalion aid stations for emergency medical and surgical care. As the patients were transported on the skids of the aircraft, medical care during transport was nonexistent. Critically ill or injured casualties were later transported to well-equipped hospital ships for definitive care and repatriation.

By 1960, the mass production of more powerful gas turbine engines allowed the design of larger, more powerful helicopters. For the first time, battlefield casualties could ride inside the helicopter and receive in-flight care from medical personnel. Medical evacuation of battlefield casualties by helicopter, often referred to as "dust off," was heavily used during the Vietnam War and was responsible for a significant improvement in the outcome of wounded soldiers. In modern warfare, medical evacuation by both helicopter and fixed-wing aircraft plays an important role in the safety of military personnel.

The civilian use of aircraft for medical evacuation and care was initiated in rural areas, such as those in Australia and Canada. Most notably, Australia developed the Royal Flying Doctor Service (RFDS) that provided medical care to the inhabitants of rural Australia. The RFDS continues to operate today. The first dedicated air ambulance service in the United States was begun by Schaeffer Ambulance Service in Los Angeles. The service opened in 1947 and was the first to use aircraft certified by the Federal Aviation Administration (FAA) in an ambulance role. By the late 1960s, the helicopter had proven itself as an effective means of transport for critically injured military casualties. However, this life-saving technology saw little, if any, use in the civilian sector.

In 1970, Congress passed legislation creating the Military Assistance to Safety and Traffic (MAST) program. This authorized the U.S. military to use the battle-proven system of simultaneous helicopter evacuation and medical care to augment existing U.S. civilian EMS. MAST programs were established at 12 active army bases, as well as several National Guard and Army Reserve installations.

In 1970, the Maryland State Police established the first nonmilitary helicopter medical evacuation program. Two years later, St Anthony's Hospital in Denver founded the first civilian helicopter EMS (HEMS) program, called Flight for Life.

©2013 Pearson Education, Inc.
*Paramedic Care: Principles & Practice, Vol. 7, 4th Ed.*

Over the next 30 years, there was a gradual, expected growth in the HEMS industry. The majority of the new programs were hospital based. In 2001, Medicare increased the reimbursement for HEMS transport, allowing a huge growth in the community-based sector of the industry. As of 2010, there were approximately 730 HEMS bases with 900 aircraft in the United States.

**4. Describe the characteristics and capabilities of fixed-wing and rotor-wing aircraft.**                                                                    **pp. 17–20**

The two types of aircraft used in air medical transport are fixed-wing aircraft (airplanes) and rotor-wing aircraft (helicopters). Fixed-wing aircraft provide comfort, speed, and significant range, especially when compared with ground ambulances. Rotor-wing aircraft can access hard-to-reach situations and provide transport that is often quicker than that available in ground ambulances. The choice of aircraft type is usually based upon the distance of transport, medical needs, patient condition, and availability.

Fixed-wing aircraft, commonly referred to as airplanes, are vehicles capable of flight that use fixed wings to generate lift. Either a turbine engine or a piston engine typically powers fixed-wing aircraft. Some turbine-powered airplanes have a propeller (turboprop) to provide propulsion, whereas others are jet powered. In the turboprop system, most of the energy derived from the turbine goes to power the propeller. In the jet propulsion system, the turbine powers a rotary air compressor that compresses incoming air and exhausts gases and ejects these via a duct. The ejected gases generated by the turbine are the propulsion used to move the aircraft.

Most air ambulances are turbine powered and usually have at least two engines. Many fixed-wing aircraft contain pressurized cabins that allow safe and comfortable travel at altitudes that are inaccessible by aircraft without a pressurized cabin. Generally speaking, fixed-wing aircraft are somewhat larger than helicopters, with many being capable of transporting several patients at the same time. Jet airplanes have a much greater range and speed than helicopters.

Helicopters, which by definition are rotary-wing aircraft, use rotating blades, referred to as a rotor, to provide lift and propulsion. The main rotor system is supplemented by a tail rotor to counteract the natural torque produced by the rotor; without the tail rotor, the cabin and fuselage would spin in the opposite direction from the main rotors. Essentially, all helicopters used in an EMS role in the United States are powered by a turbine ("jet") engine. As of 2009, 46 percent of the EMS helicopter fleet had single engines, whereas 54 percent used twin-engine aircraft. Most EMS helicopters are considered small to medium in size. Others use a larger airframe. In the United States, most EMS helicopters have a single pilot. Some medical helicopters in the United States are capable of instrument flight rule usage.

**5. Discuss limitations, concerns, and controversies about the use of air medical transport.**                                                               **pp. 21; 25–26**

Despite the potential benefits, air medical transport has its limitations. First and foremost, especially with regard to helicopter operations, flights may be impossible during periods of inclement weather. In these cases, ground transport may be the only option. The limitation of airplanes as air ambulances is that they must land and take off from established airports. Such airports are not always in close proximity to the patient or hospital. Thus, the patient must also be transported by ground ambulance to the airport to meet the aircraft, which incurs delays to definitive care.

Air medical transport is an expensive endeavor. Costs routinely exceed $10,000 to $15,000 per transport. Insurance may cover some of these costs, but it is not uncommon for patients and their families to bear the full burden if they are uninsured or underinsured. The expense derives from the high costs of aircraft maintenance, initial and recurrent training for medical and aviation crew, 24/7 staffing and availability, fuel, and insurance. Thus, it is incumbent on providers to ensure that air medical transport is used only for patients who stand to benefit from such care.

There are significant space limitations within most small to medium-sized helicopters, which are markedly smaller than even the smallest ground ambulance. In some instances, and on some airframes, the ability to carry morbidly obese patients is quite limited, not so much from the weight itself but from the girth that prevents safe loading through clam-shell doors at the rear of the fuselage. Unfortunately, our population is slowly becoming more obese. Patients who are morbidly obese unfortunately may not be candidates for air medical transport.

Even though air medical transport, especially helicopter EMS, has become a fixture in modern EMS systems, it has not been without controversy. Significant concern has been raised by many, including the National Transportation Safety Board, regarding a perceived increase in the rate and incidence of crashes involving medical helicopters.

As of 2009, there were almost 900 helicopters in service in the United States. This brisk expansion has come under increasing scrutiny in recent years, as many helicopters are based in close proximity to one another, raising significant questions of medical necessity. There has also been increasing concern about this near-exponential expansion outside the medical community. Although many of these aircraft are flying in very rural areas with long distances between the scene of an accident and the hospital, or between rural hospitals and tertiary higher-level care, many helicopter programs are being developed in areas of the country that already have adequate air medical coverage.

Another area of significant concern arose following a series of crashes in 2008 that marred the safety record of helicopter EMS. That year there were 13 accidents that resulted in 29 fatalities. This was a significant increase in the accident and fatality rate when compared with the previous year. There was also an initiative from within the air medical community to develop and embrace strategies to improve the safety of helicopter EMS. As a result, the Patient First Air Ambulance Alliance (PFAA), a grassroots organization of medical and aviation providers, was formed. The organization is committed to ensuring that critically ill and injured patients have access to the safest and highest-quality air medical system possible.

In many respects, the HEMS industry has been the beneficiary of tools developed in the military to aid its mission. Specifically, more and more programs are using night vision goggle (NVG) technology, especially for night scene responses. In the past several years, in response to accidents in which helicopters have collided with terrain, the adoption of GPS-based helicopter-specific terrain avoidance warning systems (HTAWS) and enhanced ground proximity warning systems (EGPWS), as well as radar altimeters that precisely measure the aircraft's altitude from the ground, has improved safety. Even in 2011, however, none of these tools was mandated by the FAA to be on all EMS helicopters.

Unlike the fairly heavily regulated ground EMS industry, local and state governments have little, if any, authority to regulate air ambulances. The authority to regulate operation of air ambulances (helicopter and fixed-wing) is exclusively that of the FAA. Air ambulances fall under the authority and purview of the Airline Deregulation Act, which was signed into law in 1978. As a direct result of this act, states have been prohibited from overseeing the "quality, accessibility, availability, and acceptability" of air ambulance services. This has prevented local and state governments from developing rules and regulations for air ambulance usage.

6. **Discuss the staffing and crew configurations of air medical transport craft.** pp. 25–26

The staffing and crew configuration of air ambulances varies significantly—both in the United States and around the world. In most instances, modern medical helicopters are staffed by a three-person crew consisting of the pilot and two medical providers. In some operations, two pilots are used, increasing the crew size to four.

In the United States, approximately 95 percent of HEMS programs use a crew configuration consisting of a paramedic and a nurse. However, there are multiple variations of crew staffing ranging from nurse–nurse to nurse–respiratory therapist, nurse–doctor, or two paramedics. Occasionally, in specialty care situations, specifically trained personnel, such as a pediatric respiratory therapist or a neonatal nurse, will replace one of the regular flight crewmembers. In some rare instances in the United States, certain flight programs have a nurse–physician crew configuration. Most commonly, these are emergency physicians or emergency medicine residents functioning under the direction of an attending-level emergency physician. A crew composed of a pilot and a single medical provider (nurse, paramedic, or physician) is generally inadequate except for the transport of extremely stable patients.

The physician–nurse staffing model is much more common outside the United States, including in Europe, Australia, Japan, and South Africa—where the physicians are often anesthesiologists, intensivists, emergency physicians, or general practitioners. In some helicopter EMS operations in the United Kingdom and New Zealand, ground providers will staff medical helicopters as the need arises. Typically, staffing is based on local tradition and availability. It is very much country and system specific.

©2013 Pearson Education, Inc.
*Paramedic Care: Principles & Practice, Vol. 7, 4th Ed.*

7. **Given a scenario involving air medical response, take the actions needed to ensure effective and safe ground operations.** pp. 26–30

The decision to summon a medical helicopter should be made early in scene operations. If it is later determined that the patient or patients do not require helicopter transport the inbound aircraft can be cancelled.

Provide your local HEMS with the scene location (GPS coordinates, closest city or town, actual address, well-known landmarks, etc.) and launch information (requesting agency name and contact information, local weather conditions, presence of hazardous materials, number of patients, basic medical description, etc.).

As a part of the National Incident Management System (NIMS) and the Incident Command System (ICS), a landing zone (LZ) officer should be designated. The LZ officer should coordinate the incoming aircraft operations with the incident commander (IC). The responsibilities of the LZ officer include: selection of site, site preparation, site protection and control, air-to-ground communications with incoming aircraft, and updating IC on estimated time of arrival (eta) of aircraft.

When establishing a LZ, look for an area that is (ideally) 100 feet by 100 feet square. There should be little, if any, slope to the LZ, and it should be clear of any readily visible debris or obstructions. If the area is dusty, consider wetting the area with a light water fog pattern to prevent blowing dust (brownout) from obscuring the pilot's view during landing.

Mark the LZ with cones (day) and strobes (night). As an alternative to strobes, consider laying the cones down, pointing toward the center of the LZ, with a flashlight placed inside each cone. Avoid shining lights up toward the approaching aircraft. Lights should be directed across the LZ away from the approaching aircraft. In most circumstances, the approach and landing will be made as near into the wind as practical, keeping in mind obstructions and terrain. A marker on the upwind side of the LZ (such as a cone or strobe) is conventional practice.

LZ security is of critical importance from the time of initial approach until the aircraft departs. Nonessential personnel and all vehicles and equipment must be kept clear of the LZ during this period.

Have personnel walk the LZ looking for debris, obstructions, or other dangers. The mnemonic "HOTSAW" is sometimes used to remind crews of potential hazards (hazards, obstructions, terrain, surface, animals, and wind/weather). It is also important not only to look around a LZ, but also to look up! Many forget that aircraft work in a three-dimensional environment and are of course approaching from above, so be sure to look up and assess the LZ for any obstructions above, such as wires, poles, and trees.

Ideally, during night landings, as the helicopter approaches, turn off flashing white lights (the pilot may request that other lights be turned off), use spotlights to mark any possible obstacles (e.g., overhead wires, trees, poles), and do not shine lights (or lasers) at the helicopter. Many medical helicopters use night vision imaging systems during night operations. These devices significantly increase visible light. If these are being used, the crew may request that many scene lights be turned off to ensure a safe landing.

Never allow anyone to approach the aircraft until the crew has indicated it is safe to do so. Always remain well outside the rotor perimeter and LZ until it is safe to approach (as indicated by the flight crew). The pilot may or may not leave the helicopter running. Under no circumstances should anyone approach the tail of a helicopter, even if it has a shrouded or ducted tail rotor, as it can easily be forgotten and unseen and is very dangerous.

Personnel should approach the aircraft only from the front and while in direct view of the flight crew. If the aircraft is on unlevel ground, always approach from the downhill side. Walk away from the aircraft in the same direction from which you approached it. Allow the crew to open the doors and remove any needed equipment.

Do not bring the patient directly to the helicopter. The flight crew will typically come to the patient to ensure adequate assessment and packaging for transport. After exiting the aircraft, the helicopter flight crew should be directed to the patient. The primary caregiver should give a brief, concise report of the patient's condition, describe any care provided, and detail the response to such care.

If asked to do so, assist the flight crew in loading the patient. Again, follow all safety rules for approaching and leaving the aircraft. Do not hold any equipment above shoulder height. Always follow any directions of the flight crew. Keep an eye on the crew, as verbal communications are often difficult because of the noise. Allow the crew to close and secure the doors and any outside compartments.

If an ambulance is used to move the patient to the aircraft, it should never get closer than 25 feet to the aircraft. If any vehicle contacts any portion of the helicopter or blades, that helicopter will be considered inoperable until inspected by a mechanic.

Once the crew has secured the patient, leave the LZ and remain at a safe distance. Assist the crew by being alert for open doors or compartments. Look for any straps left hanging out. Immediately notify the pilot of any new or unseen hazards. Remain in contact with the aircraft until it is well clear of the area.

8. **Given a scenario involving air medical response, obtain and communicate information needed for safe and effective interaction between the air medical crew and ground personnel.** pp. 26–30

Follow your local procedure for requesting air medical services. Provide your local HEMS with the scene location (GPS coordinates, closest city or town, actual address, well-known landmarks, etc.) and launch information (requesting agency name and contact information, local weather conditions, presence of hazardous materials, number of patients, basic medical description, etc.).

The LZ officer should remain in contact with the incoming aircraft and respond to any requests made by the pilot. Be sure the pilot is aware of specifics of the LZ, including any hazards (trees, wires, etc.).

Generally speaking, the crew of the inbound aircraft will notify you when they are close to the scene (generally 5 minutes out). In turn, notify them when you hear the aircraft and when you are able to see it. Although you can see the aircraft, its crew may not be able to see you.

If necessary to provide guidance to the approaching aircraft, use clock-based directional terms. Always consider the point of reference for the pilot (the nose of the aircraft) to be the 12 o'clock position. When the aircraft is on final approach, limit communications to safety concerns. If at any time the LZ becomes unsafe (e.g., a person wanders onto LZ), say, "Abort landing!" The LZ officer should move to a safe distance and continue to watch for hazards.

After landing, the flight crew will indicate when it is safe to approach the aircraft. After exiting the aircraft, the helicopter flight crew should be directed to the patient. The primary caregiver should give a brief, concise report of the patient's condition, describe any care provided, and detail the response to such care. Always follow any directions of the flight crew. Keep an eye on the crew, as verbal communications are often difficult because of the noise.

Once the crew has secured the patient, leave the LZ and remain at a safe distance. Assist the crew by being alert for open doors or compartments. Look for any straps left hanging out. Immediately notify the pilot of any new or unseen hazards. Remain in contact with the aircraft until it is well clear of the area.

# Case Study Review

*Reread the case study on page 15 in* Paramedic Care: Operations; *then, read the following discussion.*
*This case study draws attention to the importance of safely utilizing air medical services.*

It is vital to notify local air medical services as soon as possible, as it takes several minutes to check the weather, prepare to fly, and cover the distance to the scene of the accident. Unlike ground EMS and fire operations, which are often dispatched with an urgency that results in only seconds or minutes before they are out the door, flight crews must be careful to properly assess all the variables, such as weather, hazards, and terrain, before accepting a flight.

While care continues for the patient, other responders need to prepare for the landing, ground time, and take-off of the helicopter. Ideally, a landing zone should be 100 feet by 100 feet with little or no slope. The area should be free of debris, trees, wires, and obstructions. The LZ can be marked with cones or strobes depending on time of day and your local procedures. If the LZ is dusty, a little water fog can be used to dampen the dust; however, a charge fire hose is rarely needed during the landing, ground time, and take-off.

When the helicopter lands, ground personnel should remain in sight of the pilot and only approach when cleared to do so by the pilot or crew. Do not approach the tail rotor. It may take up to 2 minutes for the helicopter to cool down prior to shutting down. In some cases, the helicopter may not be shut down completely, commonly known as "hot loading."

©2013 Pearson Education, Inc.
*Paramedic Care: Principles & Practice, Vol. 7, 4th Ed.*

The flight crew will come to the patient and need a brief and concise report on assessment, care rendered, and response to care. The crew may complete some care, such as intubation, prior to loading the patient due to space restrictions in the helicopter.

After loading the patient, all personnel need to clear the LZ. As with the cool-down period, it may take up to 2 minutes for the helicopter to warm up prior to take-off. Most air medical services provide education to agencies about their procedures.

# Content Self-Evaluation

## MULTIPLE CHOICE

_____  1. The use of aircraft for emergency patient transport includes
   A. scene responses.
   B. interfacility transport.
   C. specialty care.
   D. organ procurement.
   E. all of the above.

_____  2. The first recorded use of an airplane to evacuate wounded casualties was during
   A. the Spanish-American War.
   B. World War I.
   C. World War II.
   D. the Korean War.
   E. the Spanish Civil War.

_____  3. In 1970, the first nonmilitary helicopter medical evacuation program was established by
   A. Loyola University Hospital in Chicago.
   B. St. Anthony's Hospital in Denver.
   C. the Los Angeles County Fire Department.
   D. the Illinois State Police.
   E. the Maryland State Police.

_____  4. Fixed-wing aircraft provide comfort, speed, and significant range, especially when compared with ground ambulances.
   A. True
   B. False

_____  5. Most EMS helicopters are considered
   A. small.
   B. small to medium.
   C. medium.
   D. medium to large.
   E. large.

_____  6. The fundamental tenets of modern trauma care introduced by Dr. R. Adams Cowley were
   A. the Golden Hour and a network of aircraft.
   B. the Platinum Ten Minutes and a network of aircraft.
   C. the Golden Hour and a network of helicopters.
   D. the Platinum Ten Minutes and a network of helicopters.
   E. the Golden Hour and a network of first-response units.

_____  7. One must not confuse the criteria for transfer to a trauma and/or burn center with the need for air transport to those facilities. Simply because a patient needs the care of a specialized center does not necessarily mean the patient must be transported by helicopter or airplane.
   A. True
   B. False

8. Limitations in using air medical transport include
   A. space limitations.
   B. high costs.
   C. high maintenance costs.
   D. inclement weather.
   E. all of the above.

9. As of 2010, there were approximately _____ HEMS bases with _____ aircraft in the United States.
   A. 530; 700
   B. 650; 800
   C. 730; 900
   D. 850; 1000
   E. 930; 1200

10. Devices that precisely measure the aircraft's altitude from the ground are
    A. enhanced ground proximity warning systems.
    B. global positioning systems.
    C. terrain avoidance warning systems.
    D. radar altimeters.
    E. none of the above.

11. The authority to regulate aviation operation of air ambulances (helicopter and fixed-wing) is exclusively that of the
    A. National Highway Traffic Safety Administration (NHTSA).
    B. U.S. Department of Transportation (USDOT).
    C. National Transportation Safety Board (NTSB).
    D. Federal Aviation Administration (FAA).
    E. State EMS agency.

12. Unlike ground EMS and fire operations, which are often dispatched with an urgency that results in only seconds or minutes before they are out the door, flight crews must be careful to properly assess all the variables, such as weather, hazards, and terrain, before accepting a flight.
    A. True
    B. False

13. Location of the scene includes
    A. well-known landmarks.
    B. GPS coordinates.
    C. closest city or town.
    D. closest cross street or roads.
    E. all of the above.

14. The responsibilities of the LZ officer include all of the following EXCEPT
    A. selection of landing zone.
    B. triage of multiple patients.
    C. communications with incoming aircraft.
    D. updating IC on aircraft ETA.
    E. landing zone protection and control.

15. The ideal landing zone is
    A. 75 feet by 75 feet, nearly level.
    B. 75 feet by 75 feet, moderate slope.
    C. 100 feet by 100 feet, nearly level.
    D. 100 feet by 100 feet, moderate slope.
    E. 150 feet by 150 feet, nearly level.

16. Generally speaking, the crew of the inbound aircraft will notify you when they are
    A. 1 minute out.
    B. 2 minutes out.
    C. 5 minutes out.

©2013 Pearson Education, Inc.
Paramedic Care: Principles & Practice, Vol. 7, 4th Ed.

**D.** 10 minutes out.

**E.** 15 minutes out.

_____ **17.** When using clock-based directional terms, the point of reference is

     **A.** the top of the aircraft.

     **B.** north.

     **C.** the tail of the aircraft.

     **D.** the nose of the aircraft.

     **E.** south.

_____ **18.** Modern turbine aircraft may take up to _____ minutes to cool down before they can be shut down.

     **A.** 1

     **B.** 2

     **C.** 3

     **D.** 4

     **E.** 5

_____ **19.** Personnel should approach the aircraft only from the rear and while in direct view of the flight crew.

     **A.** True.

     **B.** False.

_____ **20.** The paramedic should give the crew a brief, concise patient report, including

     **A.** which medications were administered.

     **B.** mechanism of injury.

     **C.** any episodes of hypotension.

     **D.** vital signs and electrocardiogram (ECG).

     **E.** all of the above.

# MATCHING

_Write the letter of the term in the space provided next to the appropriate description._

  **A.** fixed-wing aircraft

  **B.** instrument flight rules (IFR)

  **C.** night vision goggles (NVG)

  **D.** rotor-wing aircraft

  **E.** visual flight rules (VFR)

_____ **21.** Electro-optical goggles used to detect visible and infrared energy to provide a visible image in the dark

_____ **22.** Vehicles that use rotating blades (rotors) to provide lift and propulsion; helicopters

_____ **23.** Vehicles capable of flight that use fixed wings to generate lift; airplanes

_____ **24.** Regulations under which a pilot operates an aircraft in weather conditions clear enough for the pilot to see where the aircraft is going

_____ **25.** Regulations that permit an aircraft to operate in instrument meteorological conditions

# Special Project

*Identify agencies in your area that provide air medical services. Complete the following table with the agency name, contact information, and type of service (fixed-wing, rotor-wing, and if they also provide ground service). Make a copy of this table for a quick reference in your response unit.*

| AGENCY NAME | CONTACT NUMBER | TYPE OF SERVICE | | |
|---|---|---|---|---|
| | | ❑Fixed-wing | ❑Rotor-wing | ❑Ground |
| | | ❑Fixed-wing | ❑Rotor-wing | ❑Ground |
| | | ❑Fixed-wing | ❑Rotor-wing | ❑Ground |
| | | ❑Fixed-wing | ❑Rotor-wing | ❑Ground |
| | | ❑Fixed-wing | ❑Rotor-wing | ❑Ground |
| | | ❑Fixed-wing | ❑Rotor-wing | ❑Ground |
| | | ❑Fixed-wing | ❑Rotor-wing | ❑Ground |
| | | ❑Fixed-wing | ❑Rotor-wing | ❑Ground |
| | | ❑Fixed-wing | ❑Rotor-wing | ❑Ground |
| | | ❑Fixed-wing | ❑Rotor-wing | ❑Ground |

©2013 Pearson Education, Inc.
*Paramedic Care: Principles & Practice, Vol. 7, 4th Ed.*

# 3

# Multiple-Casualty Incidents and Incident Management

## Review of Chapter Objectives

### After reading this chapter, you should be able to:

1. **Define key terms introduced in this chapter.** p. 35

   Knowing and being able to apply the key terms in each chapter is critical to understanding chapter concepts. Write the list of key terms. Then write the definition of each one in your own words. Check your understanding by confirming the definitions in the text glossary. Correct any misunderstandings. Create a study aid by writing each key term on the front of an index card and the definition on the back. Use the cards to quiz yourself, or to have someone quiz you.

2. **Anticipate situations that can result in low-impact, high-impact, and disaster-related multiple-casualty incidents (MCIs).** p. 37

   **Low-Impact Incident.** A low-impact incident is one that can typically be managed by local emergency personnel. It may tax the local EMS system, but typically will not overwhelm it. Examples include a motor vehicle collision with multiple victims, a shooting with multiple victims, or similar scenarios.

   **High-Impact Incident.** A high-impact incident is one that stresses local emergency resources, including fire, police, and EMS as well as local hospitals. Examples include tornados, structural collapse, floods, and similar scenarios.

   **Disaster.** A disaster is an event that overwhelms regional emergency response resources. Examples include hurricanes, earthquakes, and major floods. Terrorist acts can also result in disaster situations.

### 3. Describe the origins and purposes of incident command or incident management systems. pp. 37–38

Based on the confusion surrounding several major fires and other large-scale incidents in the 1970s, the fire service, particularly in the Southern California area, took the lead in organizing responses to large-scale emergencies. This later evolved into a statewide system that became known as FIRE SCOPE. This system then began to be exported into other major areas around and throughout the United States. Each area had its own way of doing things and more or less adopted the basic tenets of the system that had become known as the Incident Command System (ICS).

ICS was designed for controlling, directing, and coordinating emergency response resources in as an effective manner as possible. Although the ICS was originally developed for use at major fires, a standardized ICS, or Incident Management System (IMS), has been adopted by law enforcement, EMS, hospitals, and industry.

In recent years, particularly in the months since the terrorist attacks against the United States on September 11, 2001, the various versions of the ICS or IMS in use in the United States have been merged into the comprehensive, standardized National Incident Management System (NIMS). NIMS was prescribed by way of a Homeland Security Presidential Directive (HSPD), which will, in time, require that all emergency services agencies develop and implement a comprehensive IMS that adopts the standards as prescribed by the Department of Homeland Security (DHS).

### 4. Describe the components of the National Incident Management System (NIMS). p. 39

NIMS consist of five major subsystems that collectively provide for a total system approach to all hazards and risk management.

The Incident Management System (IMS) subsystem includes operating requirements, eight interactive components, and procedures for organizing and operating an on-scene management structure.

The Training subsystem standardizes teaching that supports the effective operations of NIMS.

The Qualifications and Certification system subsystem provides for personnel across the nation to meet standard training, experience, and physical requirements to fill specific positions in the ICS.

The Publications Management subsystem includes development, publication, and distribution of NIMS materials.

The Supporting Technologies subsystem includes satellite remote imaging, sophisticated communications systems, and geographic information systems that support NIMS operations.

### 5. Describe NIMS as a uniform, yet flexible system. p. 39

With its uniform terminology and approach, the National Incident Management System has a number of advantages over the multitudes of currently existing IMSs that developed during past decades. First, NIMS recognizes that an incident can and will cross jurisdictional and geographic boundaries, and the use of a standardized and compatible management system will permit a well-organized response to routine and large-scale emergencies. Second, the NIMS has the flexibility to respond to emergencies in both the public and private sectors and incorporates concepts of business continuity and crisis management employed by the private sector to ensure the necessary continuity and continuance of critical operations.

### 6. Describe the purpose of a mutual aid coordination center (MACC). p. 39

A key element in the management of any incident that spans jurisdictions is the mutual aid coordination centers (MACCs), formerly referred to as emergency operations centers (EOCs). The MACC is a site from which civil government officials (e.g., municipal, county, state, and/or federal) exercise direction and control in an emergency or disaster. From this site, management and support personnel carry out coordinated emergency response activities.

©2013 Pearson Education, Inc.
*Paramedic Care: Principles & Practice, Vol. 7, 4th Ed.*

7. **Describe the purpose and function of each of the five major functional areas of NIMS or the Incident Command System (ICS).**

To familiarize yourself with the concepts, structure, and practices of both NIMS and the ICS, which is the fundamental tenet of NIMS, use the mnemonic C-FLOP, which stands for the first letter in each of the following functions or roles.

### Command                                                                                pp. 39–44

The most important functional area in the Incident Management System is command.

In most incidents, command is established by the first-arriving public safety official. This authority may transfer to another person based on your specific policy and procedure. Singular command is a process in which a single individual is responsible for coordinating an incident; it is most useful in single-jurisdiction incidents. Unified command is a process in which managers from different jurisdictions (law enforcement, fire, and EMS) coordinate their activities and share responsibility for command. Command is only transferred face to face, with the current IC conducting a short but complete briefing on the incident status.

### Finance/Administration                                                                 p. 45

The finance/administration section rarely operates on small-scale incidents, even though financial considerations are obviously important in all day-to-day incidents. However, on large-scale or long-term incidents, the finance/administration staff supports command by assuming responsibility for all accounting and administrative activities. This section keeps personnel and time records. It also estimates costs, pays claims, and handles procurement of items required at the incident.

### Logistics                                                                              p. 45

The logistics section supports incident operations. One of its most critical functions is operating the medical supply unit. This unit coordinates procurement and distribution of equipment and supplies at an MCI. Depending on the structure of the IMS used, other units may also be established by the logistics section. It makes sure that adequate food, water, restrooms, lighting, power, and so on are available to support incident operations.

### Operations                                                                             p. 45

Whatever work needs to be performed at an incident takes place under the operations section. This section carries out tactical objectives, directs front-end activities, participates in planning, modifies the action plan, maintains discipline, and accounts for personnel. The operations section may have many branches, which are functional levels based on primary roles or geographic locations.

### Planning/Intelligence                                                                  p. 45

The planning/intelligence section provides past, present, and future information about an incident. The planning section helps formulate the overall incident action plan (IAP) and oversees changes in that plan. It collects information such as weather reports, documents incident actions, and develops contingency plans. It ensures that written standard operating procedures (SOPs) for mutual aid agreements that govern sharing of departmental resources are activated or fulfilled. When the command and operations sections must change tactics, the planning section stands ready to provide the necessary strategic support.

8. **Describe the roles of various personnel within each of the five major functional areas of NIMS/ICS.**

### COMMAND

### Incident Commander                                                                     pp. 39–43

The incident commander (IC) is the individual who essentially runs the entire incident. The IC has the full legal authority and, in most cases, all of the associated liabilities of dealing with this incident. The IC is responsible for coordinating the many activities that occur on the emergency scene. Because it would be too confusing or impossible for all on-scene personnel to report directly to the IC, the person charged with command delegates certain functions and responsibilities to others.

On arrival, the IC will do a windshield survey of the scene. The initial size-up as well as ongoing size-ups are key in ensuring that both the operational personnel and the IC have a high level of situational awareness. During the initial and ongoing size-ups, you must keep in mind the three main priorities of all emergency services operations: life safety, incident stabilization, and property conservation.

### Safety Officer                                                                 p. 44

The safety officer (SO) may hold the most important role at an MCI. This person or, in some cases, team of people monitors all on-scene actions and ensures that they do not create any potentially harmful conditions.

### Liaison Officer                                                                 p. 44

The liaison officer (LO) coordinates all incident operations that involve outside agencies. These agencies may include other emergency services, disaster support networks, private industry representatives, government agencies, and more.

### Information Officer                                                             p. 44

The information officer (IO) collects data about the incident and releases it to the press, as well as to other agencies, on an as-needed and appropriate basis.

### Sections, Branches, Groups, Divisions, and Units                              pp. 45–49

There are several ways to divide functions at an incident. The choice of organization depends on the scope of an incident and its associated strategic goals, the structure of your department, the implementation of singular or unified command, and so on.

Command is supported by four sections or functional areas: finance/administration, logistics, operations, and planning. Each section has a place within the ICS and is headed by a section chief. All of these areas have functions that will in some way, shape, or form be fulfilled in every emergency response, even in a day-to-day-type response.

Branches may be organized by primary role or by geography. Branches are supervised by branch directors, who report to the section chief for that particular functional area.

Branches may be further organized into groups and divisions, working areas of an incident where specific job tasks are accomplished. Groups are based on function, whereas divisions are based on geography. Groups and divisions are managed by supervisors, who in turn report to the branch director.

Groups and divisions can be broken into even more task-specific groups known as units. They are supervised by unit leaders, who report to the supervisor of a group or division.

## FINANCE/ADMINISTRATION

### Finance/Administration Section                                                 p. 45

The finance/administration section rarely operates on small-scale incidents, even though financial considerations are obviously important in all day-to-day incidents. However, on large-scale or long-term incidents, the finance/administration staff supports command by assuming responsibility for all accounting and administrative activities. This section keeps personnel and time records. It also estimates costs, pays claims, and handles procurement of items required at the incident. These functions are usually performed by the jurisdictional government where the incident has occurred. The need for accuracy in the work of this unit cannot be overstressed, because a large-scale response may be eligible for reimbursements from federal or other disaster funding sources. Such reimbursements will depend directly on the ability of the agencies involved to document expenses, particularly those that are above and beyond normal operational expenditures.

## LOGISTICS

### Logistics Section                                                              p. 45

The logistics section supports incident operations. One of its most critical functions is operating the medical supply unit. This unit coordinates procurement and distribution of equipment and supplies at an

MCI. Depending on the structure of the IMS used, other units may also be established by the logistics section. The facilities unit, for example, selects and maintains areas used for command and rehabilitation. It makes sure that adequate food, water, restrooms, lighting, power, and so on are available to support incident operations. Other units might be set up to manage field communications, on-scene medical care for workers, and other functions.

## OPERATIONS

### Operations Section                                                          p. 45

Whatever work needs to be performed at an incident takes place under the operations section. This section carries out tactical objectives, directs front-end activities, participates in planning, modifies the action plan, maintains discipline, and accounts for personnel. In short, the operations section gets the job done.

As will be explained later in the chapter, the operations section may have many branches, which are functional levels based on primary roles or geographic locations. Branches organized by role might include sections within the various jurisdictions at an incident: EMS, rescue, fire, law enforcement, and so on. Branches based on geography might include operations at various locations. The IMS structure used at the 1993 bombing of the World Trade Center, for example, assigned a branch of operations to each building in the complex.

### Staging Officer                                                             p. 44

The staging officer oversees the staging area. Depending on local protocols, drivers or crew members will be required to wait with the vehicles until they are needed for transport. A staging pool keeps personnel from "freelancing" and ensures their availability for quick deployment. It also prevents premature commitment of resources.

### Triage Officer                                                              p. 46

The triage officer assumes the main responsibility for sorting patients into categories based on the severity of their injuries.

### Treatment Group Supervisor                                               pp. 52–53

The treatment group supervisor controls all actions in the treatment group/sector.

As patients arrive in the treatment area, the treatment supervisor should conduct or oversee secondary triage to determine if their status has changed.

### Morgue Officer                                                              p. 52

The morgue officer (MO) supervises the morgue. This person may report to the triage officer or the treatment officer. In many cases, these supervisors will assist in selecting and securing an area for the morgue.

### Transportation Unit Supervisor                                              p. 54

The transportation unit supervisor coordinates operations with the staging officer and the treatment supervisor. His or her job is to get patients into the ambulances and routed to hospitals. A transportation supervisor needs to implement some type of tracking system or destination log.

## PLANNING/INTELLIGENCE

### Planning/Intelligence Section                                               p. 45

The planning/intelligence section provides past, present, and future information about an incident. The planning section helps formulate the overall incident action plan (IAP) and oversees changes in that plan. It collects information such as weather reports, documents incident actions, and develops contingency plans. It ensures that written standard operating procedures (SOPs) for mutual aid agreements that govern sharing of departmental resources are activated or fulfilled.

The planning/intelligence section operates according to the principle of "anything that can go wrong will go wrong." The staff uses past incidents to anticipate trouble that might arise at the current incident. The section then acts accordingly. When the command and operations sections must change tactics, the planning section stands ready to provide the necessary strategic support.

**9. Apply a system of triage to MCIs.**                                                          **pp. 47–51**

### The START System

The most widely used triage system is START, an acronym for simple triage and rapid transport. START's easy-to-use procedures allow for rapid sorting of patients into categories. START does not require a specific diagnosis on the part of the responder. Instead it focuses on these areas: ability to walk, respiratory effort, pulses/perfusions, and neurologic status.

### The SALT System

A relatively new triage system is SALT, an acronym for sort, assess, lifesaving interventions, and treatment/ transport. SALT was developed by a working group funded by the Centers for Disease Control and Prevention (CDC) and on the best practices of major and minor triage systems in use at the time. SALT is not age specific and can be used for all age groups. Since the development of SALT, several studies have looked at the effectiveness and utility of this triage scheme. The SALT triage system has two phases: Step 1—SORT: Global Sorting; and Step 2—Assess: Individual Assessment. The SALT system is dynamic; triage assignment can be changed based on changing patient condition, scene resources, and scene safety.

### The JumpSTART System

The JumpSTART Pediatric MCI Triage Tool is an objective tool developed specifically for the triage of children in the multicasualty/disaster setting and was designed to parallel the structure of the START system, the adult MCI triage tool most commonly used in the United States. The JumpSTART system takes into consideration the anatomical and physiological differences found in children. The objectives of JumpSTART are to optimize the primary triage of injured children in the MCI setting, enhance the effectiveness of resource allocation for all MCI victims, and reduce the emotional burden on triage personnel who may have to make rapid life-or-death decisions about injured children in chaotic circumstances.

**10. Perform the various functions expected of EMS personnel in the triage, treatment, and transport branch or group in a multiple-casualty incident.**

### Triage                                                                              **pp. 46–47; 51**

Triage is the act of sorting patients based on the severity of their injuries. The objective of emergency medical services at an MCI is to do the most good for the most people. For this reason, you need to determine which patients need immediate care to live, which patients will live despite delays in care, and which patients will die despite receiving medical care. Because triage will drive subsequent incident operations, it is one of the first functions performed at an MCI.

Triage occurs in phases. Primary triage takes place early in the incident, when you first contact patients. The action provides a basic categorization of sustained injuries. It must be done quickly and efficiently so that command can determine on-site treatment needs and resources. Universally recognized triage categories include: Immediate (Red, Priority-1, P-1), Delayed (Yellow, Priority-2, P-2), Minimal (Green, Priority-3, P-3), and Expectant (Black, Priority-0, P-0).

The category names have the following meanings: *Immediate* means the patient should receive immediate treatment; *delayed* means the patient's treatment may safely be delayed; *minimal* means the patient requires minimal or no treatment; *expectant* means the patient is expected to die or is deceased.

Secondary triage is ongoing and takes place throughout the incident as patients are collected, moved to treatment areas, given appropriate medical care, and, finally, transported off scene. A patient's condition may change over time, requiring you to upgrade or downgrade his triage category.

You should attach a color-coded tag to each patient you have triaged. Tagging offers these advantages: alerts care providers to patient priorities, prevents retriage of the same patient, and serves as a tracking system during transport and/or treatment. Ideally, it will take you less than 30 seconds to triage each patient.

**Treatment**                                                                                    pp. 52–54

As patients arrive in the treatment area, you should conduct or oversee secondary triage to determine if their status has changed. Patients should then be separated into functional treatment areas based on their category. For the START Triage system: Red (Immediate, P-1), Yellow (Delayed, P-2), Green (Minimal, P-3), or Black (Expectant, P-0). For the SALT Triage system: Red (Immediate), Yellow (Delayed), Green (Minimal), Gray (Expectant), or Black (Dead).

You will also need medical equipment to operate a treatment area properly. Essential equipment includes airway maintenance supplies, oxygen and delivery devices, bleeding control supplies, and burn management supplies. In addition, you will need patient immobilization and transportation devices, such as stretchers and long spine boards.

The Red Treatment Unit provides care for all critical patients (those tagged "red"). As a result, command and/or logistics will assign the bulk of medical resources to this unit. Providers with ALS skills usually report to the red treatment area so they can stabilize patients and prepare them for transport. Because medical resources can be used up quickly, a supply system is necessary to support this operation. Finally, this is the place where any on-scene physicians or nurses should be used.

The Yellow Treatment Unit provides stabilization for all noncritical patients (those tagged "yellow"). Although these patients are not as critical as those in the red area, ALS procedures may still be necessary. A patient with an isolated femur fracture, for example, will probably be categorized yellow. Although this patient does not require immediate intervention or transport, he may still require an intravenous line and eventual surgical intervention.

The Green Treatment Unit is for ambulatory patients (those tagged "green"), where they are prepared for transport. Very little care is necessary in this area, but these patients still require monitoring in case their conditions deteriorate. In such instances, they will be retriaged and moved to the appropriate treatment area.


**Transport**                                                                                    pp. 54–55

The transportation unit supervisor coordinates transportation and will need to be flexible in determining the order in which patients are packaged and loaded. He or she may also take into account the facilities at a given hospital and avoid overwhelming its resources with critical patients.

The routing of patients to hospitals is as important as getting them into the ambulances. Early in the incident, your communications center should contact local hospitals and determine how many patients in each triage category they can handle. You must take this information into account. You must also consider any specialties that a hospital may have, such as trauma centers, burn units, and neurologic teams. Keep in mind, too, that many patients may have left the scene before the arrival of EMS and transported themselves to the closest hospital. Depending on the scope and nature of the incident, you may have to factor in such self-transport as well.

As you might suspect from this discussion, a transportation supervisor needs to implement some type of tracking system or destination log. Ideally, the tracking sheet or log will include the following data: triage tag number; triage priority; patient's age, gender, and major injuries; transporting unit; hospital destination; departure time; and patient's name, if possible. The tracking sheet not only helps to organize activities at an MCI, but it also proves invaluable in reconstructing the incident at a later time. In addition, this record will help document on-scene patient care.

11. **Describe special considerations in the response and operating
    procedures in disasters.**                                                                   p. 56

Disasters can alter the operating procedures routinely used at high-impact events.

As a rule, disaster management occurs in the following four stages: mitigation, planning, response, and recovery.

**Mitigation.** Mitigation involves the prevention or limiting of disasters in the first place. Most communities today have early-warning systems to alert people to weather emergencies, such as hurricanes and tornadoes, or to geological emergencies, such as volcanic eruptions or earthquakes.

**Planning.** Planning is integral to the successful management of all high-impact emergencies. Every community should take part in a hazard analysis and then rate these hazards according to their likelihood. Depending on the hazard analysis, devise relocation plans and/or evacuation procedures as needed.

When possible, every effort should be made to keep people in their natural social groupings. That is, provide home-based relocation instead of removing people to hospitals and clinics when they are not injured; this is commonly referred to as sheltering in place. If you must evacuate people, use whatever means you have to spread the message frequently and with urgency. Alert people to the nature of the disaster, its estimated time of impact, and provide a description of its expected severity. Advise people of safe routes out of the area and the appropriate destinations for people who must leave an area. Critical to any successful disaster plan is the provision for an efficient communications system in case the primary system fails.

**Response.** In a disaster, there is a great disparity between the casualties and resources. The event overwhelms the natural order and causes a great loss of property and/or life. As a result, a disaster almost always requires outside assistance and alternative operating plans. In general, you will follow the guidelines set up by the IMS.

**Recovery.** Recovery involves the return of your department, your jurisdiction, and your community to normal as soon as possible. Actions taken will vary with the nature of the disaster and/or the disaster plan under which you operate. You may be involved with the reunion of families, follow-up care, and support of the personnel charged with handling potential hazards such as collapsed buildings or highways.

12. **Anticipate common problems that occur in MCIs and disasters.**                    p. 57

Things can, do, and most assuredly will go wrong at MCIs and disasters. One way to avert or minimize complications is to anticipate them. Studies of past incidents have revealed the following common problems, any one of which can hinder the success of a rescue operation:

- Lack of recognizable EMS command in the field
- Failure to provide adequate widespread notification of an event
- Failure to provide proper triage
- Lack of rapid initial stabilization of patients
- Failure to move, collect, and organize patients rapidly into a treatment area
- Overly time-consuming patient care
- Premature transportation of patients
- Improper or inefficient use of in-field personnel
- Improper distribution of patients to medical facilities
- Failure to establish an accurate patient-tracking system
- Inability to communicate with on-scene units, regional EMS agencies, or other personnel
- Lack of command vests for all IMS officers or supervisors
- Lack of adequate training and/or practice of rescuers at an MCI
- Lack of drills among regional agencies involved in the IMS
- Lack of proper community assessment, preplanning, and contingency plans

13. **Describe the importance of preplanning, drills, and critiques with regard to MCI and disaster response.**                    p. 57

Planning for an MCI or disaster makes response much smoother. Anticipate any problems that may occur and work toward removing them. Anything that can be planned in advance should be planned in advance.

The first step involves a complete assessment of the potential hazards, both natural and man-made, that could occur in your area. Sites of potential incidents in almost any community include chemical or nuclear plants, factories or mines, schools, jails, sporting arenas, entertainment centers, railroads, and airports.

Once you have completed the assessment, your agency should develop a plan that outlines the SOPs and protocols for potential incidents. You will not, of course, be able to plan for every possible scenario. For this reason, you must develop contingency plans for worst-case scenarios.

After you have completed a preplan, test it. Start small. Tabletop drills, for example, are a good place to begin. Once you have worked out the wrinkles, distribute the plan to anyone who could be involved in the IMS in your area. Use the plan to ensure that the necessary mutual aid agreements are in place and that the appropriate personnel within the IMS know about these agreements.

©2013 Pearson Education, Inc.
*Paramedic Care: Principles & Practice, Vol. 7, 4th Ed.*

Then make sure that all personnel who could show up at an MCI have received proper training in use of the IMS. As you have learned, the first responders on the scene will often determine the course of an event. Run or take part in drills so that you can gain practice in MCI operations and large-scale use of the IMS. Use local drills within your department to help personnel become familiar with the system. Then, aim for large-scale drills that involve outside agencies.

Multiple-casualty incidents and disasters can occur almost anywhere and at any time. Make it part of your professional training to be ready to act as an incident commander, the person charged with establishing and organizing the IMS.

**14. Describe the role of disaster mental health services.** pp. 57–58

The emotional well-being of both rescuers and victims is an important concern in any MCI. In the past, critical incident stress management (CISM) was recommended for use in emergency services. However, recent evidence has clearly shown that CISM and critical incident stress debriefing do not appear to mitigate the effects of traumatic stress and, in fact, may interfere with the normal grieving and healing process.

Mental health personnel should be available on the scene to provide psychological first aid for those affected by the event, including emergency personnel. This requires no special training or certification and provides no psychological intervention but rather involves just meeting basic human needs, including: listening, conveying compassion, assessing needs, ensuring that basic physical needs are met, not forcing personnel to talk, providing or mobilizing company from family or significant others, encouraging but not forcing social support, and protecting from additional harm.

Competent mental health personnel can also begin to screen both rescuers and victims for abnormal signs and symptoms associated with traumatic stress.

# Case Study Review

*Reread the case study on pages 35 and 36 in* Paramedic Care: Operations; *then, read the following discussion.*

*This case study shows how, when used properly, the IMS enables EMS units to handle a multiple-patient incident without unreasonably compromising response time on other calls within the system.*

The first-arriving ambulance establishes incident command for a bus collision with 29 children and a driver. With arrival, the paramedic identifies himself as the incident commander and communicates to all the nature of the incident: "We have a school bus that veered off the road into a heavily wooded area on the shoulder of the road. Severe damage to the vehicle with a probable extrication problem. Ambulance 21 will be County Road 219 Command." This gives responding units information about the nature and scope of the incident.

In this case, the first-arriving ambulance crew locked their unit and defined their individual responsibilities as incident commander and triage officer. While the triage officer counted and tagged patients using the START system, the IC surveyed the scene for potential rescue problems, scene hazards, resource needs, and staging areas for arriving vehicles. After the triage officer reported the patient count, the IC called the dispatch center, relaying pertinent information and declaring an MCI.

The call immediately activated the regional MCI plan, proving the importance of having a plan in the first place.

Upon arrival of the field supervisor, command was transferred in a face-to-face fashion. The new IC then began setting up the various functional components required to manage the event.

Although not every community can muster multiple ambulances quickly, EMS units can still implement an IMS. Again preplanning is the key. Mutual aid agreements or broader regional plans should be in place in anticipation of worst-case scenarios. If the necessary ambulances are not readily available, operations will expand their activities in the treatment sector, while the transportation officer carefully prioritizes the routing of patients based upon available resources.

A few things that were not spelled out in the case should come to mind as you reread it. The incident commander should establish a location for an incident command post, if one is used, and mark it. Command vests are very helpful in identifying the command officers and should be used at the incident. Before establishing a staging area, command should talk with the police, especially when on a highway. The police will be responsible for traffic control as well as investigations and scene security. They will need to be involved in the plan to stage and move ambulances.

Reread the final paragraph carefully. During this event, other calls were going on in the district, including another small MCI. This underscores the need for major incidents to be handled on a separate tactical communications channel. Because of the smooth operation of the IMS, patient care was not at any time compromised—fulfilling the rationale behind adhering to a standardized IMS plan.

# Content Self-Evaluation

## MULTIPLE CHOICE

_____ 1. An emergency event that involves more patients than paramedics to provide care or ambulances to transport may be called a(n)
- A. disaster.
- B. critical incident.
- C. multiple-/mass-casualty incident.
- D. mutual aid situation.
- E. command situation.

_____ 2. Which of the following MCI classifications stresses local emergency resources, including fire, police, and EMS as well as local hospitals?
- A. Disaster
- B. High-impact incident
- C. Medium-impact incident
- D. Low-impact incident
- E. Catastrophe

_____ 3. Standards being merged into a comprehensive, standardized system for use at MCIs are being developed by
- A. the Department of Homeland Security.
- B. the Environmental Protection Agency.
- C. OSHA.
- D. the National Fire Protection Association.
- E. Firescope.

_____ 4. The most important functional area in the Incident Management System is
- A. logistics.
- B. planning.
- C. command.
- D. triage.
- E. operations.

_____ 5. On average, the span of control at an MCI is around
- A. 5.
- B. 10.
- C. 15.
- D. 20.
- E. 25.

_____ 6. At an MCI, the needs of the many usually outweigh the needs of the few.
- A. True
- B. False

_____ 7. An incident that has the potential to generate additional patients is known as a(n)
- A. open incident.
- B. MCI.
- C. closed incident.
- D. ICS.
- E. contained incident.

_____ 8. In many mass-casualty incidents, singular command is not feasible because of overlapping responsibilities or jurisdictions.
- A. True
- B. False

©2013 Pearson Education, Inc.
*Paramedic Care: Principles & Practice, Vol. 7, 4th Ed.*

_____ 9. A place where officers from various agencies can meet with each other and select a management staff is called a(n)
  A. incident command post.
  B. coordination post.
  C. incident post.
  D. Incident Management System.
  E. direct operational area.

_____ 10. The cornerstone of the Incident Management System (IMS) is
  A. leadership.
  B. utilizing singular command.
  C. having enough resources.
  D. practice and drilling.
  E. communication.

_____ 11. The primary role of the incident commander is
  A. recognizing unified command.
  B. identifying a staging area.
  C. using common terminology.
  D. the strategic deployment of all resources.
  E. directing the efficient movement of patients to the emergency department.

_____ 12. To ensure flexibility, an incident commander should radio a brief progress report every 10 minutes until the event has been stabilized.
  A. True
  B. False

_____ 13. Before command can be transferred to another leader, it is necessary to report
  A. face to face.
  B. via radio.
  C. in writing at the incident command post.
  D. via an indirect contact.
  E. none of the above—a higher-ranking officer automatically takes command upon arrival.

_____ 14. The management, or command, staff handles all of the following, EXCEPT
  A. public information.
  B. safety.
  C. triage.
  D. outside liaisons.
  E. mental health support services.

_____ 15. Under the Incident Management System, the safety officer has the authority to stop any action that is deemed as life threatening.
  A. True
  B. False

_____ 16. The person or group responsible for operating the medical supply unit is the
  A. facilities unit.
  B. liaison officer.
  C. finance/administration sector.
  D. logistics sector.
  E. planning officer.

_____ 17. Which of the following is the most task-specific section at an MCI?
  A. Branch
  B. Group
  C. Division
  D. Unit
  E. Sector

_____ 18. The term _sector_ is interchangeable for a functional or geographical area.
  A. True
  B. False

**19.** Triage that takes place after patients are moved to a treatment area to determine any changes in their status is referred to as

A. secondary triage.
B. supplemental triage.
C. sector triage.
D. delayed triage.
E. primary triage.

**20.** Under the START system, a triage officer would focus on all of the following signs and symptoms, EXCEPT

A. ability to walk.
B. respiration.
C. pulses/perfusion.
D. ability to talk.
E. neurological status.

**21.** Patients with absent radial pulses should be tagged

A. red.
B. yellow.
C. green.
D. white.
E. black.

**22.** Color-coded tags that are placed on patients that have been sorted serve to

A. track the patient.
B. prevent retriage of the same patient.
C. alert care providers to patient priorities.
D. record treatment information.
E. all of the above.

**23.** One efficient way to speed up the triage process is to

A. add extra personnel to triage.
B. not use triage tags.
C. skip the primary triage.
D. not triage the walking wounded.
E. ask the IC to assist in triage.

**24.** Which of the following functional treatment areas is included in the SALT triage system but NOT in the START triage system?

A. Red
B. Green
C. Gray
D. Black
E. Yellow

**25.** An on-scene physician may be better able to

A. perform advanced treatment in the treatment area.
B. make difficult triage decisions.
C. perform emergency surgery to extricate a patient.
D. perform advanced triage in the treatment area.
E. all of the above.

**26.** An ambulance crew that is dedicated to stand by in case a rescuer becomes ill or injured is called a _____ Team.

A. Rescue Response
B. Rehabilitation
C. Extrication
D. Rapid Intervention
E. TIP

**27.** As a general rule, disaster management occurs in which four stages?

A. Mitigation, planning, response, recovery
B. Request, response, react, recover
C. Mitigation, react, recovery, recall
D. Activation, planning, mitigation, recall
E. Planning, response, react, reassess

©2013 Pearson Education, Inc.
*Paramedic Care: Principles & Practice, Vol. 7, 4th Ed.*

_____ 28. The first step in planning for an MCI or disaster involves a complete assessment of the potential hazards.
   A. True
   B. False

_____ 29. Mental health personnel should be available on the scene of a high-impact incident to help meet the emotional needs of those affected by the incident.
   A. True
   B. False

_____ 30. Psychological first aid for those affected by the event includes
   A. ensuring that basic physical needs are met.
   B. encouraging but not forcing social support.
   C. not forcing personnel to talk.
   D. conveying compassion.
   E. all of the above.

# MATCHING

_Write the letter of the term in the space provided next to the appropriate description._

A. information officer

B. closed incident

C. planning intelligence

D. C-FLOP

E. incident command post

F. scene-authority law

G. demobilized

H. span of control

I. liaison officer

J. staff functions

_____ 31. Mnemonic for the main functional areas within the NIMS

_____ 32. Supervisory roles in the NIMS

_____ 33. Coordinates all incident operations that involve outside agencies

_____ 34. The number of people a single individual can monitor

_____ 35. Collects data about the incident and releases it to the media

_____ 36. An incident that is not likely to generate additional patients

_____ 37. Release of resources no longer needed at an incident

_____ 38. Provides past, present, and future information about the incident

_____ 39. State or local statute specifying who has authority at an MCI

_____ 40. Place where command officers from various agencies can meet

## SHORT ANSWER

*Write out the terms that each of the following acronyms stands for in the space provided.*

**41.** MCI _____

**42.** C-FLOP _____

**43.** IMS _____

**44.** START _____

**45.** SALT _____

# Special Project

*Using the EMS response units in your community, design a preplan and the administrative flowchart for a low-impact incident, high-impact incident, and disaster. If these classifications are not described in your local MCI plan, use the following patient counts:*

    Low-impact incident: 3 to 10 patients
    High-impact incident: 11 to 25 patients
    Disaster: over 25 patients

*Be sure to consider normal coverage of calls in your community as well as the need for mutual aid, if necessary.*

_____

_____

_____

_____

_____

_____

©2013 Pearson Education, Inc.
*Paramedic Care: Principles & Practice, Vol. 7, 4th Ed.*

# Rescue Awareness and Operations

## Review of Chapter Objectives

### After reading this chapter, you should be able to:

1. **Define key terms introduced in this chapter.**                                 **p. 61**

   Knowing and being able to apply the key terms in each chapter is critical to understanding chapter concepts. Write the list of key terms. Then write the definition of each one in your own words. Check your understanding by confirming the definitions in the text glossary. Correct any misunderstandings. Create a study aid by writing each key term on the front of an index card and the definition on the back. Use the cards to quiz yourself, or to have someone quiz you.

2. **Describe the concept of rescue awareness training with respect to the role of paramedics in rescue situations.**                                 **p. 63**

   In most cases, it is simply not practical to train every paramedic in the detailed knowledge or operational skills necessary for each rescue specialty. It is possible, though, to instruct paramedics in the concept of rescue and to train them to what is known as an "awareness level." Awareness training imparts enough knowledge about rescue operations to EMS personnel that they can recognize hazards and realize the need for additional expertise at the scene. Rescue involves a combination of medical and mechanical skills with the correct amount of each applied at the appropriate time.

   As first responders, paramedics should understand the hazards associated with various environments, such as extreme heat or cold, potentially toxic atmospheres, and unstable structures. They should also be able to recognize when it is safe and unsafe to access the patient or attempt a rescue. If you deem an environment safe and if you have the training to attempt a rescue, you should at least participate in the rescue under the guidance of individuals with additional expertise. You should also understand the rescue process so that you can decide when various treatments are indicated or contraindicated.

   In general, all paramedics should have the proper training and personal protective equipment (PPE) to allow them to access the patient, provide assessment, and establish incident command. The "awareness level" of rescue operations includes the following environments: surface water (e.g., "low-head" dams, flat water, moving water), hazardous atmospheres (e.g., confined spaces, trenches, hazmat incidents), highway operations (e.g., unstable vehicles, hazardous cargoes, volatile fuels), and hazardous terrains (e.g., high-angle cliffs, off-road wilderness areas).

**3. Describe the protective equipment needed by rescue and EMS personnel for a variety of rescue responses.** pp. 63–65

Without the appropriate protective gear, you will jeopardize both your own safety and the safety of the patient. Some of the equipment listed in the following sections has application in many rescue situations. Other pieces of gear are appropriate to specific environments or conditions. In all rescue environments, EMS personnel should wear highly visible clothing so they can be spotted easily. Ideally, PPE should fit the situation, but gear can be adapted, if necessary. At a minimum, you should have the following rescuer protection equipment available:

- **Helmets.** The best helmets have a four-point, nonelastic suspension system. Most of the four-point suspension helmets are designed to withstand a greater impact than the two-point system found in hard hats worn at construction sites. Avoid helmets with nonremovable "duck bills" in the back—this will compromise your ability to wear the helmet in tight spaces. A compact firefighting helmet that meets National Fire Protection Association (NFPA) standards is adequate for most vehicle and structural applications. Climbing helmets work better for confined-space and technical rescues, while padded rafting or kayaking helmets are more appropriate for water rescues.

- **Eye protection.** Two essential pieces of eye gear include goggles, which should be vented to prevent fogging, and industrial safety glasses. These should be approved by the American National Standards Institute (ANSI). Do not rely on the face shields found in fire helmets. They usually provide inadequate eye protection.

- **Hearing protection.** From a purely technical standpoint, high-quality earmuffs provide the best hearing protection. However, you must take into account other factors such as practicality, convenience, availability, and environmental considerations. In high-noise areas, for example, you might use the multi-baffled rubber earplugs used by the military or the sponge-like disposable earplugs.

- **Respiratory protection.** Surgical masks or commercial dust masks prove adequate for most occasions. These should be routinely carried on all EMS units.

- **Gloves.** Leather gloves usually protect against cuts and punctures. They allow free movement of the fingers and ample dexterity. As a rule, heavy, gauntlet-style gloves are too awkward for most rescue work.

- **Foot protection.** As a rule, the best general boots for EMS work are high-top, steel-toed, and/or shank boots with a coarse lug sole to provide traction and prevent slipping. For rescue operations, lace-up boots offer greater stability and better ankle support by limiting the range of motion. They also don't come off as easily as pull-on boots when walking through deep mud. Insulation may be useful in some colder working environments.

- **Flame/flash protection.** Every service should have a standard operating procedure (SOP) calling for the use of flame/flash protection whenever the potential for fire exists. Turnout gear, coveralls, or jumpsuits all offer some arm and leg protection and help prevent damage to your uniform. They also have the added advantage of being quick and easy to don. For protection against the sharp, jagged metal or glass found at many motor vehicle crashes or structural collapses, turnout gear generally works best. For limited flash protection, use gear made from Nomex®, PBI®, or flame-retardant cotton. For high visibility, pick bright colors such as orange or lime and reflective trim or symbols. Some services, for example, have an SOP calling for highly visible gear and/or orange safety vests to be worn during all highway operations—both day and night. Insulated gear or jumpsuits are helpful in cold environments, but they can also increase heat stress during heavy work or in situations where high ambient temperatures prevail.

- **Personal flotation devices (PFDs).** If your service includes areas where water emergencies can result, your unit should carry PFDs that meet the U.S. Coast Guard standards for flotation. They should be worn whenever operating on or around water. The Type III PFD is preferred for rescue work. You should also attach a knife, strobe light, and whistle to the PFD such that they are easily accessible.

- **Lighting.** Depending on the type and location of the rescue, you might also consider portable lighting. Many rescuers carry at least a flashlight or, better yet, a headlamp that can be attached to a helmet for hands-free operation. Consider the long-burning headlamps commonly worn by mountaineers and found through catalogs, the Internet, or climbing/camping stores.

- **Hazmat suits or self-contained breathing apparatus (SCBA).** These items should only be made available to personnel who have been trained to use them. Most services or regions have special

©2013 Pearson Education, Inc.
*Paramedic Care: Principles & Practice, Vol. 7, 4th Ed.*

hazmat units to provide the highly specialized support required at rescue situations involving toxic substances.

- **Extended, remote, or wilderness protection.** If your unit provides service to a remote or wilderness area, you might need to hike into—or even be air transported into—a rugged environment. In such cases, you would be advised to have a backcountry survival pack as part of your gear. This backpack should be preloaded with PPE for inclement weather (cold, rain, snow, wind), provisions for personal drinking water (iodine tablets/water filter), snacks for a few hours (energy gels or bars), temporary shelter (tent/tarp/bivouac sack), a butane lighter, and some redundancy in lighting in case of a light-source failure.

**4. Describe equipment and measures to protect patients in rescue situations.** p. 65

Many of the considerations for rescuer safety also apply to patients, with several significant differences. A patient protective equipment cache should include at least the following items:

- **Helmets.** Patients usually do not require the same heavy-duty helmets as rescuers. As a result, the less expensive, construction-style hard hats often provide adequate protection against minor hazards. However, if you anticipate greater danger, as in climbing or caving rescues, outfit patients with the same high-grade helmets as rescuers would use in the same or similar environments.
- **Eye protection.** Vented goggles, held in place by elastic bands, are ideal. They are not as easily dislodged as safety glasses. You might also use workshop face shields.
- **Hearing and respiratory protection.** Apply the same considerations for hearing and respiratory protection as you would for yourself. Earplugs are usually adequate.
- **Protective blankets.** You should have a variety of protective blankets to shield patients from debris, fire, or weather. Inexpensive vinyl tarps do a good job of protecting patients from water, weather, and most debris. Aluminized rescue blankets protect from fire, heat, or glass dust. Commercially available wool blankets provide excellent insulation from the cold. Plastic shielding (the kind used by landscapers) and plastic trash bags of many sizes and weights are also very useful. One 55-gallon drum liner is large enough to cover a single patient. It can serve as a disposable blanket, poncho, vapor barrier, or, in a wilderness situation, bivy sack.
- **Protective shielding.** Circumstances may call for protective equipment that is more substantial than blankets or plastic sheets. All rescue teams should be trained to use backboards and other commonly found equipment as shields to protect patients from fire, weather, falling rocks or debris, glass, or other sharp-edged objects. Shields specifically designed for a Stokes basket should be available. Keep in mind that a device that shields a patient from debris or the elements may also limit rescuers' access to the patient. The more securely you package a patient, the more difficult it will be for you to monitor him. As patient care becomes more complicated, changing patient conditions may be overlooked.

**5. Describe considerations in safety procedures in the approach to rescue situations.** p. 66

At rescue situations, all teams should have written safety procedures familiar to everyone. Contents should include sections on all types of anticipated rescues. Each section should specify required safety equipment, required or prohibited actions, and any rescue-specific modifications in assignments. SOPs should include a statement requiring that a safety officer be present and an explanation of that person's relationship to incident command. Ideally, the safety officer should be someone with the knowledge and authority to intervene in unsafe situations. This person makes the "go/no go" decision in the operation.

In addition to SOPs, an EMS unit must anticipate crew assignments and special needs before the rescue operation. This task can be done through personnel screening, careful preplanning, and regular practice of any dangerous rescue techniques that members of your unit may be trained to perform. Programs exist to identify the physical capabilities of crew members. Findings of these programs could have a significant impact on personnel assignments. In addition, psychological testing is recommended. It may even be desirable to screen for specific traits, such as phobias.

One of the most critical factors in promoting safety and operational success is preplanning. Preplanning starts with the identification of potential rescue locations, structures, or activities within your area. Effective preplanning then evaluates the specific training and equipment needed to manage each of these events. The preplan also generates ideas on efficient use of existing resources and anticipates the need for additional equipment, rescuers, and/or expertise.

Due to the intensity and length of many rescue operations, provisions must be made for the maintenance and rotation of rescue personnel. Plans should be made for "standby" or staging sites that offer protection from the weather. Sites should be away from the immediate operations area and secure from bystanders and the media. Personnel should be rotated at controlled intervals. Predetermined policies should be set regarding food and hydration of crews. On-scene diets should be high in complex carbohydrates and low in sugars and fats. Fluid replacement should consist of diluted (at least 50 percent) electrolyte solutions such as those found in sports drinks.

The preplanning should be the basis of a broader regional emergency rescue plan, to be tested and modified in practice exercises. When possible, other specialized rescue agencies, such as high-angle teams, should take part in the exercises. These "test run" scenarios will give you and other members of your unit ample opportunity to utilize the Incident Management System (IMS) as it applies to rescue situations.

**6. Describe the goals and tasks of each of the seven phases of a rescue situation.**

Like any other EMS incident, rescue operations go through phases. Although specific procedures vary from area to area and from rescue to rescue, most calls will go through seven general phases: arrival and size-up, hazard control, patient access, medical treatment, disentanglement, patient packaging, and removal/transport.

### Phase 1: Arrival and Size-Up                                            p. 67

Size-up begins with the dispatcher's call and subsequent arrival at the scene. On arrival, you or another paramedic must quickly establish medical command and appoint a triage officer. You must also conduct a rapid scene size-up, determine the number of patients, and notify dispatch of the magnitude of the event.

Now is the time to implement the IMS, any mutual-aid agreements, and the procedures for contacting off-duty personnel or backup advanced life support (ALS) units. Prompt recognition of a rescue situation and identification of the specific type of rescue are essential. Often, you must make a quick "risk-versus-benefit" analysis based on the conditions found on arrival. Be careful not to overestimate your capability to handle a rescue situation. Remember that it is always easier to send back a rescue crew than to rectify a personal tragedy caused by too few rescuers or hasty heroics. Also keep in mind the realistic time needed to access and evacuate an entrapped patient.

### Phase 2: Hazard Control                                                pp. 67–68

On-scene hazards must be identified with speed and clarity. You must often deal with these hazards before even attempting to reach the patient. To do otherwise would place you and other personnel at risk. Control as many of the hazards as possible, but don't attempt to manage any condition beyond your training or skills.

The very environment in which you stand can be risk filled. Look around to determine the possibility of lightning, avalanches, rock slides, cave-ins, and so on. Manage and minimize the risks from uncontrollable hazards as soon as possible to avoid other injuries. Ensure that all personnel, for example, wear appropriate PPE. Never forget the dangers of traffic.

A sampling of the conditions you may encounter include: poisonous or caustic substances; biological agents or germ-infected materials; swiftly moving currents, floating debris, or water contaminated with toxic agents; confined spaces such as vessels, trenches, mines, or caves; extreme heights or icy rock faces, especially in mountainous situations; and possible psychological instability.

### Phase 3: Patient Access                                                 p. 68

After controlling hazards, you will then attempt to gain access to the patient or patients. Begin by formulating a plan. Determine the best method to gain access and deploy the necessary personnel. Make sure that you take steps to stabilize the physical location of the patient.

Access triggers the technical beginning of the rescue. While gaining access, you must use appropriate safety equipment and procedures. This is the point when you and/or the incident command and

©2013 Pearson Education, Inc.
*Paramedic Care: Principles & Practice, Vol. 7, 4th Ed.*

safety officer must honestly evaluate the training and skills needed to access the patient. Untrained, poorly equipped, or inexperienced rescue personnel must not put their safety and the safety of others at risk by attempting foolhardy, heroic rescues.

During the access phase, key medical, technical, and command personnel must confer with the safety officer on the strategy they will use to accomplish the rescue. To ensure that everyone understands and supports the rescue plan, a formal briefing should be held for rescue personnel before the operation begins. Even with well-trained personnel and adequate equipment, rescue efforts can be poorly executed because team members do not understand the "big picture" or they do not know what is expected of each member of the team.

### Phase 4: Medical Treatment                                                    pp. 68–70

After devising a rescue plan, medical personnel can begin to make patient contact. In general, a paramedic has three responsibilities during this phase of the rescue operation: initiation of patient assessment and care as soon as possible; maintenance of patient care procedures during disentanglement; and accompaniment of the patient during removal and transport.

If you are treating the patient, take these actions if the conditions allow. Quickly conduct an initial assessment (mental status, ABCs, and C-spine status) on each patient. The next critical steps include rapid trauma assessment for the patient with a significant mechanism of injury, detailed physical exam, and medically oriented recommendations to the evacuation team.

Because a long time may elapse before transport, a patient's condition may change dramatically during disentanglement and removal. As a result, you should perform patient assessment with two goals in mind. First, identify and care for existing patient problems. Second, anticipate changing patient conditions, and determine the assistance and equipment needed to cope with those changes.

A final positive patient outcome may depend on initial sacrifice of definitive patient care so that the patient and rescuers can be removed from imminent danger. In such cases, rapid transport of a non-stabilized patient to a safer location may be justified by the risk of injury to the rescuers and exposure of the patient to even greater complications. Rapid movement might be required even though the transport will aggravate existing patient injuries. Generally, management for the entrapped patient has the same foundation as in all emergency care.

Specifics of patient management during a rescue often follow the same or similar protocols to those used "on the street." However, some specifics may be, or should be, significantly different. Differences result mainly from the lengthy time periods often required to access, disentangle, and/or evacuate the patient. EMS personnel are trained in rapid stabilization and transport, particularly with trauma patients. However, during a rescue mission, the desire to achieve speedy transport may be impossible to fulfill. As a result, you must be able to "shift gears" mentally to an extended care situation.

In addition to extended field time, you must be prepared to provide more in-depth psychological support for rescue patients than might otherwise be required. This is especially true in situations where a patient has already been entrapped for a considerable amount of time. Establish a solid rapport with the patient, striking up a constant and reassuring conversation.

### Phase 5: Disentanglement                                                      p. 70

Disentanglement involves the actual release from the cause of entrapment, such as the dashboard of a wrecked automobile, a concrete slab from a structural collapse, or the blocked entry to a cave. This phase may be the most technical and time-consuming portion of the rescue. If assigned to patient care during this phase of the rescue, you have three responsibilities:

- Personal and professional confidence in the technical expertise and gear needed to function effectively in the active rescue zone, sometimes referred to as the "hot zone" or "inner circle"
- Readiness to provide prolonged patient care, that is, medical support of technical efforts
- Ability to call for and/or use special rescue resources

If you or another member of the rescue team cannot fulfill these requirements, reassess available rescue personnel and call for backup. Disentanglement is not a task for persons who are claustrophobic. Disentanglement is also not a task for the squeamish.

Methods used to disentangle the patient must be constantly analyzed on a risk-to-benefit basis. You and/or other members of the rescue team must balance the patient's medical needs with such concerns as the time it will take to perform treatment, the safety of the environment, and so on. Hard treatment decisions may be faced during the disentanglement phase of the operation.

### Phase 6: Patient Packaging                                              pp. 70–71

After disentanglement, a patient must be appropriately packaged to ensure that all medical needs are addressed. You must consider such things as the means of egress, for example, a litter carry through the woods versus walking a patient out. You must also factor time based on the patient's medical conditions, for example, rapid extrication techniques versus application of a Kendrick extrication device (KED).

Some forms of patient packaging can be more complex than others, depending on the specialized rescue techniques required to extricate the patient, for example, being lifted out of a hole in a Stokes basket by a ladder truck, being vertically hauled through a manhole in a Sked® stretcher, and so on. In situations where the patient may be vertical or suspended in a Stokes basket, it is paramount that the rescuer knows how to properly package the patient to prevent additional injury.

### Phase 7: Removal/Transport                                              p. 71

Removal of the patient may be one of the most difficult tasks to accomplish or it may be as easy as placing the person on a stretcher and wheeling the stretcher to a nearby ambulance. Activities involved in the removal of a patient will require the coordinated effort of all personnel. Transportation to a medical facility should be planned well in advance, especially if you anticipate any delays. Decisions regarding patient transport—whether by ground vehicle, by aircraft, or by physical carry-out—should be coordinated based on advice from medical direction. En route to the hospital, perform the ongoing assessment, repeating vitals every 5 minutes for an unstable patient and every 15 minutes for a stable patient. Update the patient's condition and administer additional therapy per medical direction.

7. **Describe the principles and practices related to surface water rescues.**      pp. 71–76

Water emergencies are among the most common categories of rescue operations. Because people are attracted to water in such great numbers and for such a wide variety of activities, accidents can take many different forms.

Most water rescues are resolved without the involvement of EMS personnel, for example, bystanders jump into a pool to pull out a struggling swimmer or other boaters rescue someone whose canoe has overturned. However, some water emergencies require that the rescuers have special training and equipment. In such cases, the temperature and dynamics of flat or moving water place both the victim and the rescuer at high risk of entrapment.

Water rescues may involve many kinds of water bodies: pools, rivers, streams, lakes, canals, flooded gravel pits, or even the ocean. Some communities also have drainage systems that remain dry until flash floods turn them into raging rivers.

Most people who get injured or drown in these bodies of water never intended to get into trouble. But one or more factors conspire to create an emergency: The weather changes, swimmers underestimate the water's power, nonswimmers neglect to wear a PFD and fall in the water, people develop a muscle stitch or cramp while in the water, submerged debris knocks waders off their feet, boats collide, and more.

Nearly all incidents in and around water are preventable. It is important for you to become familiar with safe aquatic practices. First and foremost, know how to swim and make swimming part of your physical exercise. Second, remember that even the strongest swimmer can get into trouble. Therefore, always carry PFDs aboard your unit and always wear a PFD whenever you are around water or ice. Third, you might consider taking a basic water rescue course.

**Water Temperature.** Because the human body temperature is normally 98.6°F (37°C), almost any body of water is colder and will cause heat loss. Water temperature in smaller bodies of water varies widely with the seasons and the amount of runoff. Yet, even on warm days, water temperature can be quite cold in most places. As a result, water temperature and heat loss figure in the demise of most victims and ill-equipped rescuers.

As implied, immersion can rapidly lead to hypothermia. As a rule, people cannot maintain body heat in water that is less than 92°F (33°C). In fact, water causes heat loss 25 times faster than the air. Immersion in 35°F (1.6°C) water for 15 to 20 minutes is likely to kill a person. Factors contributing to the demise of a hypothermic patient include: incapacitation and an inability to self-rescue; inability to follow simple directions; inability to grasp a line or flotation device; and laryngospasm (caused by sudden immersion) and greater likelihood of drowning.

A number of actions can delay the onset of hypothermia in water rescues. The use of PFDs slows heat loss and reduces the energy required for flotation. If people suddenly become submerged, they can also assume the heat escape lessening position (HELP). HELP can reduce heat loss by almost 60 percent, as compared to the heat expended when treading water. If a group of victims find themselves in the water, researchers also suggest huddling together. This technique not only prevents heat loss, but provides a better target (more visibility) for members of a rescue team.

**Basic Rescue Techniques.** Basic rescue techniques vary with the dynamics of the water; rescue in moving water will differ from rescue in nonmoving (flat) water. If your unit responds to frozen bodies of water, you may also add techniques for ice rescue and include the proper cold water entry dry suits as part of your PPE cache. Also keep in mind that a PFD is useless if it is not worn—all EMS personnel should put one on, even for shore-based rescues.

The water rescue model is reach–throw–row–go. All paramedics should be trained in reach-and-throw techniques. If, at first, you are unable to talk the patient into a self-rescue, then reach with a pole or long rescue device. If this is not effective or if the victim is too far out, try throwing a flotation device. Boat-based techniques require specialized rescue training. Water-entry ("go") is used only as the last resort, and is an action best left to specialized water rescuers.

**Moving and Flat Water.** By far the most dangerous water rescues involve water that is moving. Competency at handling the power and dynamics of swift-water rescues comes only with extensive training and experience. The force of moving water can be very deceptive. The hydraulics of moving water change with a number of variables, including water depth, velocity, obstructions to flow, changing tides, and more. Only specially trained rescuers can readily recognize these factors. The greatest problem with flat water is that it looks so calm. Yet, a large proportion of drowning or near-drowning incidents take place in flat or slow-moving water.

**Factors Affecting Survival.** A number of factors help determine the demise or survival of a patient. A person's "survivability profile" is affected by age, posture, lung volume, water temperature, and more. Two especially important factors include the presence of PFDs and what is known as the "cold-protective response."

**Personal Flotation Devices.** Many recreational water users associate "life preservers" with rough water or people who can't swim. But PFDs should be essential items for all water-related activities. Every system should have a strict standard operating procedure (SOP) mandating the use of PFDs for all EMS personnel. Even services in arid regions can be involved in water rescues. They can be called to swimming pool incidents or river-rafting accidents. In some places, especially in the southwest, they can respond to flash-flooding in canyons that can trap or kill hikers or "canyoneers." The same flash flooding can overload drainage systems, creating hazardous conditions for the public and rescuers alike.

**Cold-Protective Response.** Brain cells deprived of oxygen will normally begin to die in as little as 4 to 8 minutes. Keeping the head above water, as in the HELP and self-rescue techniques, ensures that the person can breathe and keep the brain supplied with oxygen. Additionally, although cold water can cause death from hypothermia, cold water can also trigger a protective response known as the "mammalian diving reflex." This is how it works: When the face of a human, or any mammal, is plunged into cold water less than 68°F (20°C), the parasympathetic nervous system is stimulated. The heart rate rapidly decreases to a bradycardic rhythm. Meanwhile, blood pressure drops and vasoconstriction occurs throughout the body. Blood is shunted from less vital organs to the heart and brain, temporarily delivering life-sustaining oxygen. As a general rule, the colder the water, the more oxygen is diverted. As a rule, the reflex is more pronounced in children than in adults.

**Location of Submerged Victims.** Because of protective physiological responses, rescuers must make every effort to locate submerged victims. Interview witnesses to establish the most accurate "last seen" location. Start searching from this point and fan out in larger and larger circles, forming a radius equal to the depth of the water.

**Rescue vs. Body Recovery.** A number of conditions determine when a rescue turns into a body recovery. Some factors are length of time submerged, any known or suspected trauma, age and physical condition of the victim, water temperature and environmental conditions, and estimated time for rescue or removal.

Once a patient is recovered, you should attempt resuscitation on any hypothermic and/or pulseless, nonbreathing patient who has been submerged in cold water. A patient must be rewarmed before an accurate assessment can be made. Remember: Water-rescue patients are *never dead until they are warm and dead.*"

**In-Water Patient Immobilization.** In flat water where you are able to safely stand, it is important that you know how to perform in-water immobilization. Cervical spine injuries are associated with trauma (e.g., diving) rather than simple submersion. In general, the procedure mirrors the application of a long board, with the following modifications: hold the patient's head in place by using the patient's arms as a "splint" (head-splint technique) and submerge the board under the patient's waist and allow the board to float up to the victim. (If the board does not float, lift it gently to the victim.)

8. **Describe special considerations and hazards for moving water rescues.** pp. 72–74

By far the most dangerous water rescues involve water that is moving. Competency at handling the power and dynamics of swift-water rescues comes only with extensive training and experience. The force of moving water can be very deceptive. The hydraulics of moving water change with a number of variables, including water depth, velocity, obstructions to flow, changing tides, and more. Only specially trained rescuers can readily recognize these factors.

To train for swift-water entry, rescuers must develop a proficiency in many specialized skills. In preparation for technical rope rescues, they must master the skills required for high-angle rope rescues. They must also become well practiced in such skills as crossing moving bodies of water, defensive swimming, use of throw bags and boogy boards, shore-based swimming, boat-based rescue techniques, management of water-specific emergencies, and the capability to package the patient with water-related injuries.

**Recirculating Currents.** Recirculating currents result from water flowing over a uniform obstruction such as a large rock or low-head dam. The movement of currents can create what is known as a "drowning machine." On first appearance, recirculating currents can look very tame. Once caught in the recirculating currents, people find it very difficult to escape. The resulting rescue can be extremely hazardous, even for specially trained rescuers.

**Strainers.** When moving water flows through obstructions such as downed trees, grating, or wire mesh, an unequal force is created on the two sides of the so-called "strainers." Currents can literally force a patient up against a strainer, making it difficult to remove him due to the power of the current. In some cases, the current might be flowing into a drainage pipe under the surface, which is in turn covered by a rebar (metal) grate. Victims can get sucked into the grate and then pinned against it.

This too can be a hazardous rescue. If you get stuck floating downstream and see the potential of getting pinned against a strainer, attempt to swim over the object. Whatever you do, don't put your feet on the bottom of the river—your feet could get stuck or, even worse, you could get swept off your feet and slammed into the obstruction.

**Foot/Extremity Pins.** It is always unsafe to walk in fast-moving water over knee depth because of the danger of entrapping a foot or extremity. When this occurs, the weight and force of the water can knock you below the surface of the water. To remove the foot or extremity, it must be extracted the same way it went in. Water currents often make this extremely difficult. Again, this is a hazardous rescue because of the need to work below the surface in already dangerous water conditions.

**Dams/Hydroelectric Intakes.** Yet another dangerous situation involves dams and hydroelectric intakes, such as those often found along rivers. The height of the dam is no indication of the degree of hazard. As a result, assume that all dams have the ability to form recirculating currents. Hydroelectric intakes, however, serve as dangerous strainers with all the accompanying hazards.

**Self-Rescue Techniques.** If you suddenly fall in moving or flat water keep these suggestions in mind:
- Wear an appropriate PFD.
- Use the HELP and HUDDLE positions.
- Cover your mouth and nose during entry.
- Protect your head and, if possible, keep your face out of the water.
- Do not attempt to stand up in moving water.
- Float on your back, with your feet pointed downstream.
- Steer with your feet, and point your head toward the nearest shore at a 45-degree angle or continue to float downstream until you come to an area where the water slows enough for you to swim to the edge.
- If the water turns a bend, remember that the outside of the curve moves faster that the inside of the curve.
- Look for large objects, such as rocks, that can block the water and cause recirculating currents or strainers.
- Learn to identify eddies—water that flows around especially large objects and, for a time, flows upstream around the downside of the obstruction.
- Above all else, take precautions not to fall into the water in the first place. Remember: Reach–throw–row–go, with "go" being the absolutely last resort.

9. **Describe the principles and practices related to hazardous atmosphere rescues.** pp. 76; 78–79

Confined-space rescues present any number of potentially fatal threats, but one of the most serious is an oxygen-deficient environment. At first glance, most confined spaces appear relatively safe. As a result, you might mistakenly think rescue procedures will be easier and/or less time consuming and dangerous than they really are. Examples of confined spaces are transport or storage tanks, grain bins and silos, wells and cisterns, manholes and pumping stations, drainage culverts, pits, hoppers, underground vaults, and mine or cave shafts.

Confined spaces present a wide range of hazards. You may confront one or more of these hazards in any given confined-space rescue. As a first responder, it is your responsibility to identify these hazards as soon as possible, both for purposes of scene safety and for summoning the necessary support. Some of the most common risks include the following: oxygen-deficient atmospheres, toxic or explosive chemicals, engulfment, machinery entrapment, electricity, and structural concerns.

The types of confined-space emergencies most commonly encountered in the workplace include falls, medical emergencies (often hazmat related), oxygen deficiencies or asphyxia, explosions, and entrapment. You should never allow rescuers into a confined space unless they have the training, equipment, and experience specific to the particular environment involved. You will almost always summon outside specialized agencies for support.

If a collapse has caused burial, a secondary collapse is likely. Therefore, your initial actions should be geared toward safety. Secure the scene, establish command, secure a perimeter, and immediately summon a team specializing in trench rescue. While waiting for the team to arrive, do not allow entry in the area surrounding the trench or cave-in. Safe access can take place only when proper shoring is in place.

10. **Describe the principles and practices related to highway operations and vehicle rescues.** pp. 80–84

The most common rescue situations encountered by EMS personnel involve motor vehicle collisions. These incidents generally go through the phases covered at the start of this chapter. However, certain modifications must be made to meet the special hazards associated with traffic control and the extrication of patients from wrecked vehicles.

To prepare for highway rescues, you must size up the scene, identify all hazards, and ensure scene safety by controlling any potentially dangerous situations. In the case of highway operations, this means reducing traffic-related hazards and identifying hazards related to the vehicle crash itself.

In managing highway operations or vehicle rescues, you should use the following general strategies: initial scene size-up, control hazards, assess the degree of entrapment and fastest means of extrication, establish circles of operation, and treatment, packaging, and removal of the patient.

Depending on local protocols, you should practice or observe the use of the rescue skills and equipment needed for initial vehicle stabilization. You should also make a point of practicing and/or observing the various disentanglement or extrication skills commonly used with vehicle rescues, many of which have already been mentioned. Know how to gain access using hand tools through nondeformed doors, deformed doors, safety and tempered glass, trunks, and floors. Become familiar with the use of heavy hydraulic equipment employed by special rescue teams in your area and take part in practice scenarios to build agency cooperation. Preplan and prepare so that you are ready when this all-too-common type of rescue occurs.

**Traffic Hazards.** Traffic flow is the largest single hazard associated with EMS highway operations. You may have to respond to incidents on roads with limited access and to incidents on highways with unlimited access. In either situation, you will need to work closely with police to avoid unnecessary congestion as well as other injuries. An even bigger personal danger results from the risk of vehicles hitting EMS apparatus or personnel. At this point in your career, you probably already know some of the things you can do to reduce traffic hazards. A few tried-and-tested techniques include: staging, positioning of apparatus, emergency lighting, redirection of traffic, and high visibility.

**Other Hazards.** Other hazards besides traffic control exist at highway operations. In some communities, paramedics receive training to manage these hazards. In other communities, they receive "awareness training" and learn to summon specialized rescue personnel. Regardless of the procedure in your service area, you must be able to recognize all nontraffic hazards. Otherwise, you risk injuring yourself, your crew, the patient, or even passing motorists. Some of these nontraffic hazards include: fire and fuel, alternative fuel systems, hybrid and electric vehicles, sharp objects, electric power, energy-absorbing bumpers, supplemental restraint systems (SRSs)/air bags, hazardous cargoes, rolling vehicles, and unstable vehicles.

**Auto Anatomy.** Motor vehicle collisions present EMS personnel with the most common access and/or extrication problems. As a result, you must know some basic information about automobile construction or "anatomy." Obviously, vehicles can differ greatly, both in terms of manufacture and design. However, most recent automobiles have certain features in common that can guide you in simple access situations.

Vehicles can have either a unibody or a frame construction. For unibody vehicles to maintain their integrity, all of the following features must remain intact: roof posts, floor, firewall, truck support, and windshield.

Both types of construction have roofs and roof supports. The support posts are lettered from front to back. The first post, which supports the roof at the windshield, is called the "A" post. The next post is the "B" post, and so on. If you remove the plastic molding on the posts, the remaining steel can be easily cut with a hacksaw. In the case of a unibody design, remember that cutting a post will interrupt the vehicle's construction.

The firewall separates the engine compartment and the occupant compartment. The firewall can collapse on a patient's legs during a high-speed head-on collision. Movement at other parts of the vehicle, such as cutting a rocker panel or roof support post, can place additional pressure on the feet.

The engine compartment usually contains the battery. This can cause a fire hazard; therefore, many rescue teams cut the battery cables to eliminate this risk. Before disconnecting the power, it is a good idea to move back electric seats and lower power windows. Otherwise, you might needlessly complicate the extrication.

Vehicles have two types of glass: safety glass and tempered glass. Safety glass is found in windshields and is designed to stay intact when shattered or broken. However, safety glass can still produce glass dust or fracture into long shards. These materials can easily get into a patient's eyes, nose, or mouth and/or create cuts. As a result, be sure to cover a patient whenever you remove this type of glass. Tempered glass has a high tensile strength. However, it does not stay intact when shattered or broken. It fractures into many small beads of glass, all of which can cause injuries and cuts.

Before attempting to assist a patient through a door, you should be trained in proper extrication techniques. Try all four doors first; otherwise, gain access through the window farthest away from the patient(s). Alternatively, use simple hand tools to peel back the outer sheet of metal on the door, exposing the lock mechanism. Unlock the lock and pry the cams from around the Nader pin. Then pry out the door.

©2013 Pearson Education, Inc.
*Paramedic Care: Principles & Practice, Vol. 7, 4th Ed.*

**Hybrid Vehicles.** Hybrid automobiles, also called hybrid electric vehicles (HEVs), contain both an electric motor and an internal combustion motor. A large array of batteries powers the electric motor while the internal combustion motor is powered by gasoline or diesel fuel. The electrical system of HEVs contains a high-voltage component and a 12-volt battery. The high-voltage component poses a particular risk for rescue personnel. The easiest way to inactivate the high-voltage component is to simply turn off the vehicle and remove the key from the ignition. This prevents electric current from flowing into the cables from the motor or high-voltage battery, and turns off power to the airbags and the seat belt pre-tensioners. To assure rescuer safety, it is recommended that the 12-volt battery also be disconnected to further isolate the electrical system. Because battery locations vary by vehicle type, rescuers should be familiar with the popular HEV vehicle types on the market.

**11. Describe the principles and practices related to hazardous terrain rescues.**                                             pp. 84–87

As a paramedic, you must know how to take part in rugged terrain rescues. At a minimum, you should know how to perform litter evacuations without causing additional injury to patients. Even more important, you should develop a "rescue awareness" so that you know when to call specialized teams and how to work with those teams once they arrive on the scene.

Low-angle terrains typically can be accessed by walking or scrambling—climbing over boulders or rocks using both hands and feet. Footing can be difficult, and it may be hazardous to carry a litter even with multiple people. As a result, low-angle teams use ropes to counteract gravity and/or may set a rope to act as a hand line. Any error can result in a fall or tumble. Depending on the presence of boulders, brush, downed trees, and so on, injuries can be quite serious.

High-angle terrain usually involves a cliff, gorge, side of a building, or terrain so steep that hands must be used when scaling it. Crews depend on rope and/or aerial apparatus for access and litter movement. Errors are likely to cause serious, life-threatening injuries. In many cases, falls can be fatal.

Flat terrain with obstructions includes trails, paths, and creek beds. Obstructions can take many forms, such as downed trees, rocks, slippery leaves or pine needles, and scree—the loose pebbles or rock debris that can form on the slopes or bases of mountains. Although this is the least hazardous type of rugged terrain, it is still possible to slip while carrying a patient, causing injury.

Unless you have been trained in high-angle or low-angle rescue, patient access and removal should be left to specialized teams. Even if you have the skills to perform the rescue, you will in all likelihood need additional resources to provide the necessary balance of technical and medical support for the patient.

Depending on local protocols, you should practice the packaging and evacuation techniques expected of EMS personnel in your region. You should familiarize yourself with the specific types of basket stretchers and litters available to your unit and the proper packaging, immobilization, and restraint techniques for use with each type. You should also practice with other equipment used for rough terrain rescues, including the Sked® and appropriate half-spine devices. Practice or observe the skills required for low-angle and high-angle rescues. When possible, take part in exercises with the rescue units that you would summon to perform these evacuations. By fully understanding the capabilities of the rescue response teams in your area, you will know how to work together whenever a multi-jurisdictional event occurs.

**High-Angle Rescues.** High-angle, or vertical, rescuers must constantly contend with the effects of gravity. Any organization that could be assigned a vertical technical rescue must have extensive initial training, additional advanced training, frequently supervised practice sessions, and top-of-the-line equipment. Each member of a high-angle team must have complete competency in knot tying, use of ladders and/or ropes to ascend and descend a steep face, ability to rig a hauling system, and the skills for packaging a patient for evacuation by litter and rope. Some of the specialized terms that you will hear high-angle rescuers use include: aid, anchor, belay, and rappel.

**Low-Angle Rescues.** Many EMS systems have trained their paramedics in the skills of low-angle rescue or "off-the-road" rescue. Like high-angle rescues, crews require rope, harnesses, hardware, and the necessary safety systems. A rescue is considered a low-angle rescue up to 40°, except if the face is overly smooth. In that case a high-angle team will be better able to handle the more technical access and evacuation.

Each member of a low-angle crew must know how to assemble a hasty harness tied from 2-inch tubular webbing (or don a climbing harness), rappel and ascend by rope, package a patient in a litter, and rig a simple hauling system to assist the litter team up the embankment. Teams must also know how to set up a hasty rope slide to assist with balance and footing on rough terrain. Although low-angle rescues involve less technical skill than high-angle rescues, they still require ongoing practice and proper equipment.

**Patient Packaging for Rough Terrain.** Packaging a patient is a critical aspect of any hazardous terrain rescue. The Stokes basket stretcher is the standard litter for rough terrain evacuation. Alternative spinal immobilizers can be used in a Stokes basket such as the KED, "halfback" backboard (extrication/rescue vest), or the Sked®. As a last resort, the Stokes itself can be used as a spinal immobilizer. Plastic basket stretchers are usually weaker than their wire mesh counterparts. However, they tend to offer better patient protection. In general, Stokes baskets with plastic bottoms and steel frames are best. These versatile units can also be slid in snow, when necessary.

Most Stokes baskets are not equipped with adequate restraints, and thus they will require additional strapping or lacing for rough terrain evacuation and/or extrication. A plastic litter shield can be used to protect the patient from dust and objects that may fall on the person's face.

**Patient Removal from Hazardous Terrain.** When removing the patient from hazardous terrain, a nontechnical/nonrope evacuation is usually faster. In other words, when possible, walk the patient out. Carrying a patient on a litter over flat ground can be a strenuous task even under ideal conditions. As the terrain becomes rougher, the litter carry becomes more demanding.

When removing a patient in a litter from flat, rough terrain, make sure you have enough litter carriers to "leapfrog" ahead of each other to save time and to rotate rescuers. An adequate number of litter bearers would be two or, better yet, three teams of six. Litter bearers on each carry should be approximately the same height.

Low-angle and high-angle evacuations require specialized knowledge and skills. Before beginning patient removal, rescuers must ensure that all anchors are secure. They must check their own safety equipment and recheck patient packaging. They must also have the necessary lowering and hauling systems in place, again doing the recommended safety checks.

Materials, especially ropes, should never be used if there is any question of their safety. If you see a frayed rope or any stressed or damaged equipment, do not hesitate to point it out to the rescuers in a polite, but professional manner. Also, because hauling sometimes requires many "helpers," you may be asked to assist. Make sure you understand all directions given by the rescuers. Evacuation is a team effort.

Some high-angle units, especially within fire departments, make use of aerial apparatus such as tower-ladders or bucket trucks to assist in the removal of a patient in a Stokes basket. These units are usually employed in structural environments, but can be adapted to hazardous terrain if there is room for a truck. When using aerial apparatus, it is necessary to provide a litter belay during movement to a bucket. Litters, of course, must then be correctly attached to the bucket. Use of aerial ladders can be difficult because the upper sections are usually not wide enough to slot the litter. The litter must always be properly belayed if being slid down the ladder. Finally, ladders or other aerial apparatus should NOT be used as a crane to move a litter. They are neither designed nor rated for this work. Serious stress can cause accidents resulting in patient death.

**Use of Helicopters.** Helicopters can be useful in hazardous terrain rescues, especially when hospitals lie at a distant location. You must understand the capabilities of local helicopter systems and know who provides helicopter rescue in your region. Be aware of the difference in mission, crew training, and capabilities of helicopters that do air medical care versus helicopters that do rescue.

12. **Describe considerations for extended care of patients in rescue situations.** p. 87–88

For rescue operations, at least some personnel should have formal training in managing patients whose injuries have been aggravated by prolonged lack of treatment, often under extreme conditions. If SOPs do not already exist, procedures adopted from wilderness medical research will prove useful. Position papers written by the Wilderness Medical Society or the National Association for Search and Rescue can serve as guidelines for protocols. If your agency anticipates involvement in some of the rescue

©2013 Pearson Education, Inc.
*Paramedic Care: Principles & Practice, Vol. 7, 4th Ed.*

situations described in this chapter, you should consider protocols that at least address the following areas:

- Long-term hydration management
- Repositioning of dislocations
- Cleansing and care of wounds
- Removal of impaled objects
- Nonpharmacologic pain management
- Pharmacologic pain management
- Assessment and care of head and spinal injuries
- Management of hypothermia or hyperthermia
- Termination of cardiopulmonary resuscitation (CPR)
- Treatment of crush injuries and compartment syndrome

A number of environmental issues can affect your assessment during a rescue situation. Some of the most important issues include the following: weather/temperature extremes, limited patient access, difficulty transporting street equipment, cumbersome PPE, patient exposure, use of ALS skills, patient monitoring, and improvisation.

Whatever you do, continue talking to the patient and explain exactly what is happening. Answer any questions, particularly if you are improvising. The patient is already frightened by the entrapment. Don't worsen the situation by making the patient feel even more out of control.

# Case Study Review

*Reread the case study on page 62 in* Paramedic Care: Operations; *then, read the following discussion.*

*The case study emphasizes the importance of rescue awareness and the cooperative effort that takes place between medical and technical crews.*

It was critical that the rescue team immediately called for specialized resources, in this case a high-angle team and helicopter. As indicated, it takes time for these resources to arrive on-scene and, once there, even more time to reach and package the patient. It would have helped if more EMS teams had been sent in for backup. For example, additional personnel could have helped in carrying the Stokes litter to the helicopter. Even the short distance of 200 yards can be a difficult carry for two people.

Fortunately, the patient was removed before the storm hit. However, if the storm had come in faster, the helicopter might not have been able to make the call. In such an instance, many rescuers would have been required to access the patient, now exposed to severe environmental conditions. They also would have faced evacuation during a storm. Don't be surprised if a helicopter is not always able to respond to your call for assistance. Plan for the worst-case scenario. As stressed in this chapter, "Don't undersell overkill."

# Content Self-Evaluation

## MULTIPLE CHOICE

_____ 1. As applied to rescue operations, awareness training involves a(n)
   A. command of the technical skills to execute a rescue.
   B. ability to recognize hazards.
   C. realization of the need for additional resources.
   D. detailed knowledge of rescue specialties.
   E. both B and C.

_____ 2. Most PPE used in rescue situations has been designed for the field of EMS.
   A. True
   B. False

3. The person(s) who makes a "go/no go" decision in a rescue operation is the
   A. medical dispatcher.
   B. incident commander.
   C. specialized rescue crew.
   D. safety officer.
   E. first responders.

4. In what phase of a rescue operation does patient access take place?
   A. First
   B. Second
   C. Third
   D. Fourth
   E. Fifth

5. The technical phase of a rescue begins with
   A. scene size-up.
   B. medical treatment.
   C. access.
   D. hazard control.
   E. packaging.

6. During an extended rescue, take all the following steps to calm patient fears, EXCEPT to
   A. explain all delays.
   B. tell the patient you will not abandon him.
   C. minimize the dangers of the situation.
   D. explain unfamiliar technical aspects of the operation.
   E. be sure the patient knows your name.

7. Water causes heat loss 25 times faster than the air.
   A. True
   B. False

8. Actions to delay the onset of hypothermia in water rescues include all of the following, EXCEPT
   A. use of PFDs.
   B. use of HELP.
   C. huddling together.
   D. treading water.
   E. both C and D.

9. The first action you should take in a water rescue is to
   A. reach for the patient with a pole.
   B. swim to the patient.
   C. row to the patient.
   D. throw a flotation device to the patient.
   E. talk the patient into a self-rescue.

10. At a low-head dam, one of the biggest dangers to rescue is a(n)
    A. strainer.
    B. foot pin.
    C. recirculating current.
    D. eddy.
    E. large rocks.

11. Factors that affect the survival of a patient in a drowning incident include
    A. age.
    B. lung volume.
    C. water temperature.
    D. posture.
    E. all of the above.

12. You should attempt resuscitation on any hypothermic and/or pulseless, nonbreathing patient who has been submerged in cold water.
    A. True
    B. False

13. The primary reason confined spaces present a potentially fatal threat is because
    A. a patient cannot get out and panics.
    B. of a lack of OSHA regulations.
    C. the space is oxygen deficient.
    D. of faulty retrieval devices.
    E. none of the above.

©2013 Pearson Education, Inc.
*Paramedic Care: Principles & Practice, Vol. 7, 4th Ed.*

14. Although all of the following present risks, the largest single hazard associated with EMS highway operations is
    A. sharp objects.
    B. traffic flow.
    C. rollover situations.
    D. hazardous cargoes.
    E. alternative fuel systems.

15. The easiest means of accessing a motor vehicle patient is through the
    A. windshield.
    B. door.
    C. window closest to the patient.
    D. hatch.
    E. rear window.

16. Removal of the patient from the vehicle almost always precedes patient care.
    A. True
    B. False

17. The easiest way to inactivate the high-voltage component in a hybrid vehicle is to
    A. turn off the vehicle.
    B. remove the key from the ignition.
    C. disconnect the 12-volt battery.
    D. turn off the vehicle and remove the key from the ignition.
    E. disconnect the high-voltage battery.

18. The LEAST important skill for a member of a high-angle rescue team is
    A. rappelling.                          D. anchoring.
    B. scrambling.                          E. rigging a hauling system.
    C. belaying.

19. Most Stokes stretchers are NOT equipped with adequate restraints.
    A. True
    B. False

20. Which of the following probably would NOT be found in a downsized backpack?
    A. SAM splints                          D. Intubation equipment
    B. Small oxygen tank/regulator          E. Extrication collars
    C. ECG monitor

# MATCHING

*Write the letter of the term in the space provided next to the appropriate description.*

A. recirculating currents

B. mammalian diving reflex

C. extrication

D. come-along

E. eddies

F. HELP

G. safety glass

H. active rescue zone

 I. short haul

 J. tempered glass

_____ 21. Area where special rescue teams operate

_____ 22. Use of force to free a patient from entrapment

_____ 23. An in-water, head-up tuck or fetal position designed to reduce heat loss

_____ 24. Movement of currents over a uniform obstruction

_____ 25. Type of glass with a high tensile strength that fractures into small beads when shattered

_____ 26. Helicopter extrication technique where a person is attached to a rope that is, in turn, attached to a helicopter

_____ 27. Ratcheting cable device used to pull in a straight direction

_____ 28. Water that flows around especially large objects and, for a time, flows upstream on the downside of the object

_____ 29. A type of glass made from three layers of fused materials that is designed to stay intact when shattered

_____ 30. The body's natural response to submersion in cold water, the end process of which increases blood flow to the heart and brain

# Special Project

## Specialized Mechanical Support

_Check with your service chief or an EMS director to find out which special rescue units or teams you would call for backup in each of the following types of emergencies. Record the information in the spaces below._

**Vehicle Rescue**

Name: _____

Contact number: _____

Services provided: _____

_____

_____

_____

**Swift-Water Rescue**

Name: _____

Contact number: _____

Services provided: _____

**High-Angle Rescue**

Name: _____

Contact number: _____

Services provided: _____

_____

_____

_____

**Ice Rescue**

Name: _____

Contact number: _____

Services provided: _____

_____

_____

_____

**Confined-Space Rescue**

Name: _____

Contact number: _____

Services provided: _____

_____

_____

_____

**Trench Rescue**

Name: _____

Contact number: _____

Services provided: _____

_____

_____

_____

# Hazardous Materials

## Review of Chapter Objectives

### After reading this chapter, you should be able to:

**1. Define key terms introduced in this chapter.**                                    **p. 92**

Knowing and being able to apply the key terms in each chapter is critical to understanding chapter concepts. Write the list of key terms. Then write the definition of each one in your own words. Check your understanding by confirming the definitions in the text glossary. Correct any misunderstandings. Create a study aid by writing each key term on the front of an index card and the definition on the back. Use the cards to quiz yourself, or to have someone quiz you.

**2. Describe the distribution of hazardous materials throughout the country.**        **p. 93**

Hazardous materials (hazmats) are all around us. Companies in the United States manufacture more than 50 billion tons of hazardous materials a year. Some 4 billion tons of hazardous materials are shipped throughout the United States by truck, pipeline, railroad, and tankers. They can exist as solids, liquids, or gases. They can irritate, burn, poison, corrode, or asphyxiate.

   According to the U.S. Department of Transportation (DOT), a hazardous material can be regarded as "any substance which may pose an unreasonable risk to health and safety of operating or emergency personnel, the public, and/or the environment if not properly controlled during handling, storage, manufacture, processing, packaging, use, disposal, or transportation."

**3. Relate your training in response to toxicological emergencies, multiple-casualty incidents, and terrorism to the response to hazardous materials.**        **pp. 93–96**

As you know from Volume 4, Chapter 8: Toxicology and Substance Abuse, a person can be exposed to a hazardous substance in four ways: inhalation, absorption, injection, or ingestion. The most common method is respiratory inhalation. In hazmat situations, the least common route of exposure is through gastrointestinal ingestion, but it does happen. In occupations involving hazardous materials, people can be exposed to poisons by eating, drinking, or smoking around deadly substances. Foodstuffs can be exposed to a chemical and then eaten. People can forget to wash their hands and introduce the substance into their mouths.

   Priorities for a hazmat incident are the same as those for any other major incident: life safety, incident stabilization, and property conservation. In setting priorities, you must also quickly determine whether the hazmat emergency is an open incident or a closed incident. That is, does the event have the potential for generating more patients? As you learned in Chapter 3: Multiple-Casualty Incidents and Incident Management, the answer to this question will determine the resources that you request, how you stage them, and the way in which you deploy personnel. In reaching your decision, remember that some chemicals have delayed effects. Triage must be ongoing, because patient conditions can change rapidly. Finally, in employing the Incident Management System (IMS) at a hazmat incident, you must take into account certain special conditions when choreographing the scene. The basic IMS at a hazmat incident will require a command post, a staging area, and a decontamination corridor. Depending on the event, the incident commander may also establish separate areas, such as treatment areas and personnel staging areas, to prevent unnecessary exposure to contamination.

Unfortunately, a new type of hazmat incident has emerged in the form of terrorism. Terrorists may use any variety of chemical, biological, or nuclear devices to strike at government or high-profile targets. These weapons of mass destruction (WMDs) can be manufactured from materials as simple as those found on most farms. The most frightening aspect of terrorism is the lack of predictability about when or where an attack might take place. Lacking a clear verbal or written threat, it can happen almost anyplace anywhere. See Chapter 8: Responding to Terrorist Acts for additional information.

In responding to a suspected terrorist incident, look for potential clues. Patients in a closed environment, such as a subway or an office building, will exhibit similar symptoms if they have been exposed to a chemical or biological WMD. In the case of an explosion, remember that a secondary device may exist. Take every precaution not to fall victim to a terrorist attack yourself. Make full use of the IMS and all specialized agencies able to respond to the scene of suspected terrorism.

4. **Describe the need for specialized training at various levels to effectively manage hazardous materials incidents.** **p. 94**

Two federal agencies, the Occupational Safety and Health Administration (OSHA) and the Environmental Protection Agency (EPA), have set forth a number of regulations and standards for dealing with hazmat emergencies. The most important of these are found in OSHA publication CFR 1910.120, *Hazardous Waste Operations and Emergency Response Standard* (2004). This standard provides specific response procedures, including use of an IMS, use of personal protective equipment (PPE), use of a safety officer, and special training requirements. The EPA has published a mirror regulation, 40 CFR 311, that applies to those agencies that fall outside of OSHA's jurisdiction. In addition, the National Fire Protection Association (NFPA) has published NFPA 473, *Standard Competencies for EMS Personnel Responding to Hazardous Materials Incidents*. This standard, along with two other NFPA standards for hazmat response, deals with the training standards for EMS personnel assigned to hazmat incidents.

The awareness level applies to responders who may arrive first at a scene and discover a toxic substance. Training focuses on recognition of hazmat incidents, basic hazmat identification techniques, and individual protection from involvement in the incident. All EMS personnel, as well as police officers and firefighters, need to be trained to the Awareness Level.

EMS Level 1 training, or the "operations level," is required for those who may perform patient care in the cold zone on patients who do not present a significant risk of secondary contamination. This training focuses on hazard assessment, patient assessment, and patient care for previously decontaminated patients.

EMS Level 2 training, or the "technician level," is required for those who may perform patient care in the warm zone on patients who still present a significant risk of secondary contamination. This training focuses on personal protection, decontamination procedures, and treatment for patients who are beginning or undergoing decontamination.

The level of training required for each individual depends on that person's role in the hazmat response system. All systems require some individuals to be trained in both the EMS Level 1 and Level 2 standard. In this way, patient care can begin during decontamination and continue after the patient has been cleaned of contaminants.

5. **Describe the paramedic's role at hazardous materials incidents.** **pp. 93–94**

Hazardous materials incidents, or hazmat incidents, present some of the most challenging situations that you will face as a paramedic. Traditionally, paramedics do not perform defensive (containment) and offensive (control) functions at a hazardous materials response. Even so, paramedics are still an integral part of a community's hazmat response system.

EMS personnel fulfill a variety of tasks at a hazmat incident. As first responders, they may size up the incident, assess the toxicological risk, and activate the IMS needed to handle the event. They will

©2013 Pearson Education, Inc.
*Paramedic Care: Principles & Practice, Vol. 7, 4th Ed.*

also be called on to evaluate decontamination methods, to treat and transport exposed patients, and to perform medical monitoring of hazmat teams that enter the area.

**6. Recognize situations that may involve a hazardous material release.** pp. 93–94

Hazardous materials may be spilled or released as a result of an accident, equipment failure, human error, or an intentional violation of the laws and regulations that govern their manufacture, use, and disposal.

A hazmat event can involve all kinds of substances: corrosive chemicals, pulmonary irritants, pesticides, chemical asphyxiants, hydrocarbon solvents, and radioactive wastes. The exposure to hazardous materials may be limited to just a few victims, or it may cause widespread destruction and loss of many lives.

**7. Given a variety of scenarios involving hazardous material release, identify the substance and use resources to determine information about the substance and actions to take.** pp. 96–99

Once you have determined that an incident involves hazardous materials, you must next try to identify the particular substance. This is the "crux," or most difficult aspect, of dealing with a hazmat incident. You will often lack adequate on-scene information to make a positive identification, or you will get conflicting preliminary information. For this reason, you must be familiar with the resources that can assist you in identification of a hazardous material and become skilled at using each of them. To prevent dangerous interpretations, try to locate two or more concurring reference sources. Do not take action until you find this information, otherwise you risk making mistakes and providing incorrect patient treatment.

**Placards.** Placards are easily spotted because of their diamond shape. Each placard indicates hazmat classifications through use of a color code and hazard class number. Some placards also carry a UN number specific to the actual chemical. In addition to numbers and colors, placards also use symbols to indicate hazard types. When combined with numbers and colors, these symbols help you to recognize the specific nature of the hazardous material.

Although some substances are required to show a placard in any quantity, others need to be placarded only if they are transported in large quantities. This means that a truck may be carrying hazardous materials, but because the amount falls below the quantity required for placarding, no placard is shown. Also, the "Dangerous" placard means that there are two or more substances on board between 1,000 and 5,000 pounds total weight. However, the generic placard tells you nothing about the hazardous nature of the materials. Finally, people can remove placards or fail to apply them in the first place. In this case, you have no immediate indication at all of a dangerous hazmat situation.

**NFPA 704 System.** The NFPA 704 System identifies hazardous materials at fixed facilities. Like the DOT placards, the system uses diamond-shaped figures, which are placed on tanks and storage vessels. The diamond is divided into four sections and color coded. The top segment is red and indicates the flammability of the substance. The left segment is blue and indicates the health hazard. The right segment is yellow and indicates the reactivity. The bottom segment is white and indicates special information. The information may include water reactivity, oxidizing capability, or radioactivity. Flammability, health hazard, and reactivity are measured on a scale of 0 to 4. A designation of 0 indicates no hazard, whereas a designation of 4 indicates extreme hazard.

***Emergency Response Guidebook.*** The *Emergency Response Guidebook* (ERG), published by the U.S. Department of Transportation, Transport Canada, and the Secretary of Communications and Transportation of Mexico, should be carried on every emergency vehicle. It lists more than a thousand hazardous materials, along with placards, UN numbers, and chemical names. It also cross-references each identification number to specific emergency procedures related to the chemical. The ERG includes, for example, a list of evacuation distances for the most hazardous substances. It is revised frequently, and the most up-to-date version should be readily available to all crew members.

When using the ERG, keep in mind two shortcomings. First, the reference provides only basic generic information on medical treatment. Second, more than one chemical often have the same

UN number. The difference between these chemicals can be dramatic, highlighting the need to use other methods of positive identification.

**Shipping Papers.** The most accurate information about a transported substance can be found in the shipping papers, or bill of lading. Trucks, boats, airplanes, and trains routinely carry these documents. Ideally, they should list the specific substances and quantities carried. However, drivers, pilots, or engineers may not take these papers when they exit the vehicle or craft, and you may find the scene too unstable to retrieve the documents yourself. In some cases, the papers may be incomplete or inadequate, requiring you to consult additional sources of identification.

**Material Safety Data Sheets (MSDSs).** In the case of fixed facilities, employers are required by law to post material safety data sheets (MSDSs). These sheets contain detailed information about all potentially hazardous substances found on the site. The sheets typically list the names and characteristics of the materials; what types of health, fire, and reactivity dangers the materials pose; any specific equipment or techniques required for safe handling of the materials; and suggested emergency first-aid treatment.

Even simple chemicals, such as window cleaners, should have MSDSs posted in an easily accessible location. Among other information, the MSDS indicates possible adverse reactions in cases of accidental exposure, spills, leaks, and so on.

**Monitors and Testing.** If you are unable to secure positive identification using other sources, you may have to rely on monitors and other means of testing. If you do not have the training and equipment to do the reconnaissance, leave testing to the hazmat team. Monitoring devices or materials typically include: air and gas monitors (percentage of oxygen in the air and measure the presence of explosive gases, carbon monoxide, and toxic gases), litmus paper (approximate pH of a liquid, indicating whether it is an acid or a base), and colormetric tubes (air sampling for specific chemicals).

**Other Sources of Information.** Once you have identified the hazardous substance, you will need to determine its specific chemical or physical properties. You can consult textbooks, handbooks, or technical specialists. You might also make use of a computerized database such as Computer-Aided Management of Emergency Operations (CAMEO®). Another source of information is your local or regional poison control center.

Two other sources of information are the Chemical Transportation Emergency Center (CHEMTREC) and CHEMTEL. CHEMTREC maintains a 24-hour, toll-free hotline. It provides information on the chemical properties of a substance and explains how the material should be handled. If necessary, CHEMTREC will even contact shippers and manufacturers to find out more detailed information about the incident and provide field assistance. CHEMTEL, Inc., maintains another 24-hour, toll-free emergency response communications center for the United States and Canada. In addition to providing support for chemical emergencies, CHEMTEL also supplies the names of state and federal authorities that deal with radioactive incidents.

8. **Describe the various control zones established at a hazardous materials incident.** p. 101

**Hot (Red) Zone.** The hot zone, also known as the exclusionary zone, is the site of contamination. Prevent anyone from entering this area unless they have the appropriate high-level PPE. Hold any patients that escape from this zone in the next zone, where decontamination and/or treatment will be performed.

**Warm (Yellow) Zone.** The warm zone, also called the contamination reduction zone, lies immediately adjacent to the hot zone. It forms a "buffer zone" in which a decontamination corridor is established for patients and EMS personnel leaving the hot zone. The corridor has both a "hot" and a "cold" end.

**Cold (Green) Zone.** The cold zone, or "safe zone," is the area where the incident operation takes place. It includes the command post, medical monitoring and rehabilitation, treatment areas, and apparatus staging. The cold zone must be free of any contamination. No people or equipment from the hot zone should enter until they have undergone the necessary decontamination. You and your crew should remain inside this zone unless you have the necessary training, equipment, and support to enter other areas.

©2013 Pearson Education, Inc.
*Paramedic Care: Principles & Practice, Vol. 7, 4th Ed.*

### 9. Take actions to protect yourself and other responders from exposure at the scene of a hazardous materials incident. pp. 99; 101–108

Your main priority at a hazmat incident is safety. First, you protect your own safety and the safety of your crew. Then you attend to the safety of the patient(s) and the public.

Prepare for the arrival of additional resources by setting up the control zones: hot (red or exclusionary) zone, warm (yellow or contamination reduction) zone, and cold (green or safe) zone.

Whenever people or equipment come into contact with a potentially toxic substance, they are considered to be contaminated. The contamination may be either primary or secondary. Primary contamination occurs when someone or something is directly exposed to a hazardous substance. At this point, the contamination is limited—that is, the exposure has not yet harmed others. Secondary contamination takes place when a contaminated person or object comes in contact with an uncontaminated person or object—that is, the contamination is transferred. If you touch a contaminated patient, for example, you can become a contaminated care provider. Although gas exposure rarely results in secondary contamination, liquid and particulate matter are much more likely to be transferred.

The PPE used at a hazmat incident is specifically designed to prevent or limit rescuer injuries. Hard hats, for example, protect rescuers against impacts to the head. There are basically four levels of hazmat protective equipment, ranging from Level A (the highest level) to Level D (the minimum level). The level of hazmat protective gear worn depends on the chemical or substance involved. All ambulances carry some level of PPE, even if not ideal. If the situation is emergent and the chemical unknown, use as much barrier protection as possible. Full turnout gear (Level D) or a Tyvek suit is better than no gear at all. High-efficiency particulate air (HEPA) filter masks and double or triple gloves offer good protection against some hazards. Keep in mind that latex gloves are not chemically resistant. Instead, use nitrile gloves, which have a high resistance to most chemicals. Also remember that leather boots will absorb chemicals permanently, so be sure to don rubber boots.

The decontamination method and type of PPE depend on the substance involved. If in doubt, assume the worst-case scenario. When dealing with unknowns, do not attempt to neutralize. Brush dry particles off the patient before the application of water to prevent possible chemical reactions. Next, wash with great quantities of water—the universal decon agent—using a tincture of green soap if possible. Isopropyl alcohol is an effective agent for some isocyanates, and vegetable oil can be used to decon water-reactive substances. Use the two-step decon process for gross decontamination of patients who cannot wait for a more comprehensive decon process. The eight-step process takes place in a complete decontamination corridor and is much more thorough.

When transporting field-decontaminated patients, always recall that they may still have some contamination in or on them. As a result, use as much disposable equipment as possible. Keep in mind that any airborne hazard can not only incapacitate the crew in the back of the ambulance, but can affect the driver as well.

### 10. Describe the levels of hazardous materials protective equipment available. pp. 108–109

Personal protective equipment used at a hazmat incident is specifically designed to prevent or limit rescuer injuries. There are basically four levels of hazmat protective equipment, ranging from Level A (the highest level) to Level D (the minimum level).

**Level A.** Provides the highest level of respiratory and splash protection. This hazmat suit offers a high degree of protection against chemical breakthrough and fully encapsulates the rescuer, even covering the self-contained breathing apparatus (SCBA). The sealed, impermeable suits are typically used by hazmat teams entering hot zones with an unknown substance and a significant potential for both respiratory and dermal hazards.

**Level B.** Offers full respiratory protection when there is a lower probability of dermal hazard. The Level B suit is nonencapsulating, but chemically resistant. Seams for zippers, gloves, boots, and mask interface are usually sealed with duct tape. The SCBA is worn outside the suit, allowing increased maneuverability and greater ease in changing SCBA bottles. The decon team typically wears Level B protective equipment.

**Level C.** Includes a nonpermeable suit, boots, and gear for protecting the eyes and hands. Instead of SCBA, Level C protective equipment uses an air-purifying respirator (APR). The APR relies on filters to protect against a known contaminant in a normal environment. As a result, the canisters in the APR must be specifically selected and are not usually implemented in a hazmat emergency response. Level C clothing is usually worn during transport of patients with the potential for secondary contamination.

**Level D.** Consists of structural firefighter, or turnout, gear. Level D gear is usually not suitable for hazmat incidents.

The level of hazmat protective gear worn depends on the chemical or substance involved. Ideally, the chemical should be identified so a permeability chart can be consulted to determine the breakthrough time. No single material is suitable to all hazmat situations. Some materials are resistant to certain chemicals and nonresistant to others.

**11. Describe approaches to decontaminating patients exposed to a variety of hazardous materials.** p. 106

The four methods of decontamination are dilution, absorption, neutralization, and isolation/disposal. The method used depends on the type of hazardous substance and the route of exposure. In many instances, rescuers will use two or more of these methods during the decontamination process.

**Dilution.** Dilution involves the application of large quantities of water to the contaminated person or item. Water is considered the universal decon solution, especially for reducing topical absorption. It may be aided by use of a soap, such as a tincture of green soap. Mixing hazardous substances with water significantly reduces their concentration, hopefully to a level at which they are no longer dangerous. Be aware that a small number of chemicals should never be mixed with water.

**Absorption.** Absorption entails the use of pads or towels to blot up the hazardous material. The process is usually applied after washing with water—that is, as a means of drying the patient. Absorption further reduces the contamination levels but is not usually a primary method of decon. Absorption is more commonly used during environmental cleanup.

**Neutralization.** Neutralization occurs when one substance reduces or eliminates the toxicity of another substance, such as adding an acid to a base. Although this is a third method of patient decontamination, it is almost never used by EMS personnel. In a field setting, it is difficult to identify the exact hazardous substance and the proper neutralizing agent. In addition, neutralization often produces an exothermic reaction, or release of large quantities of heat. The heat can be just as damaging as, or even more damaging than, the original chemical. Lavage usually dilutes and removes the chemical faster and is more practical given the typical on-scene equipment.

**Isolation/Disposal.** Isolation and/or disposal involves separating the patient or equipment from the hazardous substance. Isolation begins by establishing zones at the incident to prevent any further contamination or exposure. Next, hazmat teams remove patients from the hot zone to the warm zone. Last, any items that might contain or trap a hazardous substance should be removed, including a patient's clothing and jewelry. All contaminated items should be properly disposed of or stored.

**12. Given a variety of hazardous materials scenarios, demonstrate safe and effective patient care.** pp. 104–105

Patients can be exposed to an incredibly large number of chemicals. Their treatment ranges from supportive care to specific antidotes. After ensuring your own safety, you should see that all patients receive the necessary supportive measures: airway support and suctioning, respiratory support, supplemental oxygen, circulatory support, and intravenous access. Before administering specific pharmacologic treatment, at least two sources should agree on the medication. In addition, you should confer with medical direction.

**Corrosives.** Corrosives (acids and alkalis) can be found in many everyday materials. Corrosives can be inhaled, ingested, absorbed, or injected. Primary effects include severe skin burns and respiratory burns and/or edema. Some corrosives may also have systemic effects. When decontaminating a patient exposed to solid corrosives, brush off dry particles. In the case of liquid corrosives, flush the exposed area with large quantities of water. A tincture of green soap may help in decontamination. Irrigate eye injuries with water, possibly using a topical ophthalmic anesthetic such as tetracaine to reduce eye discomfort. In patients with pulmonary edema, consider the administration of furosemide (Lasix) or albuterol. If the patient has ingested a corrosive, DO NOT induce vomiting. If the patient can swallow and is not drooling, you may direct the person to drink 5 mL/kg water up to 200 mL. As with other injuries, maintain and support the ABCs: airway, breathing, and circulation.

**Pulmonary Irritants.** Many different substances can be pulmonary irritants. Primary respiratory exposure cannot be decontaminated. However, you should remove the patient's clothing to prevent any trapped gas from being contained near the body. You should also flush any exposed skin with large quantities of water. Irrigate eye injuries with water, possibly using tetracaine to reduce eye discomfort. Treat pulmonary edema with furosemide, if indicated. Again, treatment includes maintaining and supporting the ABCs.

**Pesticides.** Toxic pesticides or insecticides include primarily carbamates and organophosphates. Patients may come in contact with these chemicals through any of the four routes of exposure: inhalation, absorption, ingestion, or injection. The substances can act to block acetylcholinesterase (AChE), an enzyme that stops the action of acetylcholine, a neurotransmitter. The result is overstimulation of the muscarinic receptors and the SLUDGE syndrome: salivation, lacrimation, urination, diarrhea, gastrointestinal distress, and emesis. Stimulation of the nicotinic receptor may also trigger involuntary contraction of the muscles and pinpoint pupils.

These chemicals will continue to be absorbed as long as they remain on the skin. As a result, decontamination with large amounts of water and a tincture of green soap is essential. Remove all clothing and jewelry to prevent the chemical from being trapped against the skin. Maintain and support the ABCs. Secretions in the airway may need to be suctioned.

The primary treatment for significant exposure to pesticides is atropinization. The dose should be increased until the SLUDGE symptoms start to resolve. For carbamates, pralidoxime is NOT recommended. If an adult patient presents with seizures, administer 5 to 10 mg of diazepam. Do NOT induce vomiting if the patient has ingested the chemical.

**Chemical Asphyxiants.** The most common chemical asphyxiants include carbon monoxide (CO) and cyanides such as bitter almond oil, hydrocyanic acid, potassium cyanide, wild cherry syrup, prussic acid, and nitroprusside. Keep in mind that both CO and cyanides are by-products of combustion, so patients who present with smoke inhalation may need to be assessed for these substances as well. Most patients are exposed to CO and cyanides through inhalation. However, keep in mind that cyanides can also be ingested, absorbed, or injected.

These two chemicals have different actions once inhaled. Carbon monoxide has a very high affinity for hemoglobin—approximately 200 times greater than that of oxygen. As a result, it displaces oxygen in the red blood cells. Cyanides, however, inhibit the action of cytochrome oxidase. This enzyme complex, found in cellular mitochondria, enables oxygen to create the adenosine triphosphate (ATP) required for all muscle energy. Primary effects of CO exposure include changes in mental status and other signs of hypoxia such as chest pain, loss of consciousness, or seizures. Primary effects of cyanides include rapid onset of unconsciousness, seizures, and cardiopulmonary arrest.

Decontamination of patients exposed to CO and cyanide asphyxiants is usually unnecessary. However, these patients must be removed from the toxic environment without exposing rescuers to inhalation. Take off the patient's clothing to prevent entrapment of any toxic gases, while maintaining airway, breathing, and circulatory support. Definitive treatment for CO inhalation is oxygenation. In some cases, it may be provided through hyperbaric therapy, which increases the displacement of carbon monoxide from hemoglobin molecules by oxygen. Definitive treatment for cyanide exposure can be provided by one of two cyanide antidotes.

The older system, generally referred to as a cyanide antidote kit (also called a Pasadena, Lilly, or Taylor kit), contains three medications: amyl nitrite, sodium nitrite, and sodium thiosulfate. If this kit is used, first administer amyl nitrite. This short-acting vasodilator has the ability to convert hemoglobin to methemoglobin, which forms a nontoxic complex with cyanide ions. Wrap an ampule in gauze or cloth and crush it between your fingers. Then place it in front of a spontaneously breathing patient for 15 seconds. Repeat at 1-minute intervals until an infusion of sodium nitrite is ready. Keep in mind that amyl nitrite is volatile and highly flammable when mixed with air or oxygen. Next, administer the sodium nitrite, 300-mg IV push over 5 minutes. (Sodium nitrite also produces methemoglobin.) Quickly follow the sodium nitrite with an infusion of sodium thiosulfate, 12.5-g IV push over 5 minutes. The sodium thiosulfate converts the cyanide/methemoglobin complexes into thiocyanate, which can be excreted by the kidneys. If the signs and symptoms reappear, the process should be repeated at half the original doses.

A safer and less toxic antidote is now available. This antidote, called hydroxocobalamin, is commercially available and packaged as Cyanokit™. Hydroxocobalamin is a precursor to cyanocobalamin (vitamin $B_{12}$). When hydroxocobalamin is administered, it binds cyanide from cytochrome oxidase and forms cyanocobalamin. Excess cyanocobalamin is excreted from the body via the kidneys.

**Hydrocarbon Solvents.** Many different chemicals can act as solvents, including xylene and methylene chloride. Usually found in liquid form, they give off easily inhaled vapors. Primary effects include dysrhythmias, pulmonary edema, and respiratory failure. Delayed effects include damage to the central nervous system and the renal system. Exposure to these chemicals may be intentional, such as among drug abusers seeking the central nervous system effects (euphoria) produced by the fumes. If the patient ingests the chemical and vomits, aspiration may lead to pulmonary edema. Treatment varies with the route of exposure. In cases of topical contact, decontaminate the exposed area with large quantities of warm water and a tincture of green soap. If the patient has ingested the solvent, DO NOT induce vomiting. If the adult patient presents with seizures, administer 5 to 10 mg of diazepam. In the case of inhalation, maintain and support the ABCs.

13. **Describe the role of EMS personnel in monitoring and rehabilitation of those responding to a hazardous materials incident.** pp. 109–110

One of the primary roles of EMS personnel at a hazmat incident is the medical monitoring of entry personnel. All hazmat team members should undergo regular annual physical examinations, with baseline vital signs placed on file.

Prior to entry, you or other EMS crew members will assess rescuers and document the following information on an incident flow sheet: blood pressure, pulse, respiratory rate, temperature, body weight, electrocardiogram (ECG), and mental/neurologic status. If you observe anything abnormal, do not allow the hazmat team member to attempt a rescue.

The PPE used at hazmat incidents can cause significant stress and dehydration. As a result, entry team personnel should prehydrate themselves with 8 to 16 ounces of water or sport drinks. Because sport drinks are more effective at half strength, dilute them with 50 percent water when possible.

After the hazmat entry team members exit the hot zone and complete decontamination, they should report back to EMS for post-entry monitoring. Measure and document the same parameters on the flow sheet. Rehydrate the team with more water or diluted sports drinks. You can use weight changes to estimate any fluid losses. Check with medical direction or protocols to determine fluid replacement by means of PO or IV. Entry team members should not be allowed to reenter the hot zone until they are alert, nontachycardic, normotensive, and within a reasonable percentage of their normal body weight.

In evaluating heat stress, you will need to take many factors into account. Primary considerations include temperature and humidity. Prehydration, duration and degree of activity, and the team member's overall physical fitness will also have a bearing on your evaluation. Keep in mind that Level A suits protect a rescuer, but prevent cooling. A rescuer essentially works inside an encapsulated sauna. The same suit that seals out hazards also prevents heat loss by evaporation, conduction, convection, and radiation. Therefore, place heat stress at the top of your list of tasks for post-exit medical monitoring.

# Case Study Review

*Reread the case study on pages 92 and 93 in* Paramedic Care: Operations; *then, read the following discussion.*

This case study presents the decisions facing paramedics summoned to the scene of a chemical burn incident. Fortunately, a plant supervisor is able to identify the hazardous material. Remember, however, that this is not always the case, and you will have to try to determine the substance before approaching the scene.

Even if the paramedics know nothing about the incident, patient symptoms provide a clue to the presence of a hazardous material. Although it is not unusual to respond to a call with multiple patients, it is noteworthy when all of the patients exhibit similar symptoms, in this case shortness of breath. Whenever you

©2013 Pearson Education, Inc.
*Paramedic Care: Principles & Practice, Vol. 7, 4th Ed.*

arrive at a scene to find multiple patients with similar medical complaints, suspect that they have been exposed to a hazardous material. The most common toxic inhalant is carbon monoxide from a faulty heating system in a residence. Treat similar symptoms as a "red flag."

As with most hazmat incidents, the team immediately initiates the Incident Management System. Other steps that might have been taken in the initial stages of the incident would include donning appropriate PPE and, perhaps, looking up the properties and recommended treatment for anhydrous ammonia in one of the references mentioned in this chapter (or consulting with medical direction).

Important points in the case include the use of gross contamination, efforts to relocate all personnel away from the runoff (to avoid further contamination), and the way in which the EMS crew interacted with the hazmat team, including the appropriate pre- and post-monitoring steps.

In this case, treatment was provided. However, this should only be done after ensuring your own safety and conferring with medical direction to avoid any synergistic complications.

# Content Self-Evaluation

## MULTIPLE CHOICE

1. Which first responders need to be trained to the hazmat awareness level?
   A. All EMS personnel
   B. Police officers
   C. Firefighters
   D. A and C
   E. A, B, and C

2. Upon arriving at the scene of a potential hazmat incident, the first step you should take is to
   A. size up the scene.
   B. don PPE.
   C. activate the IMS.
   D. refer to OSHA CFR 1910.120.
   E. establish command.

3. The most preferable site for deploying resources at a hazmat scene is
   A. uphill and downwind.
   B. uphill and upwind.
   C. across the street from the incident.
   D. 1 mile away.
   E. 100 yards away.

4. The basic IMS at a hazmat incident will require all of the following, EXCEPT a
   A. staging area.
   B. decontamination corridor.
   C. transport zone.
   D. command post.
   E. treatment area.

5. One of the most critical aspects of any hazmat response is
   A. working with unified command.
   B. establishing the time the incident began.
   C. transporting all patients who have been exposed.
   D. the awareness that a dangerous substance is present.
   E. treating critically injured patients.

6. A diamond-shaped graphic placed on vehicles to indicate hazard classification is a(n)
   A. placard.
   B. MSDS.
   C. UN number sign.
   D. NFPA label.
   E. ERG.

7. One of the most difficult aspects of dealing with a hazmat incident is
   A. reading hazmat references.
   B. identifying the particular substance.
   C. working with uncooperative patients.
   D. establishing EMS command.
   E. communicating with the media.

8. Shipping papers that contain accurate information about a transported substance are known as
    A. transport vouchers.
    B. MSDSs.
    C. bills of lading.
    D. cargo filings.
    E. special protection information.

9. Data sheets containing detailed information about all potentially hazardous substances found at a work site are called
    A. placards.
    B. MSDSs.
    C. UN number signs.
    D. NFPA labels.
    E. reactivity data sheets.

10. Hazmat monitoring devices should be routinely used by EMS personnel for quick identification of a substance.
    A. True
    B. False

11. Which safety zone is also called the contamination reduction zone or buffer zone?
    A. Hot zone
    B. Warm zone
    C. Cold zone
    D. Treatment zone
    E. Extrication zone

12. Which of the following is (are) LEAST likely to result in secondary contamination?
    A. Acids and alkalis
    B. Carbon monoxide
    C. Organophosphates
    D. Liquid corrosives
    E. Carbamates

13. In hazmat situations, the least common route(s) of exposure is (are) through
    A. respiratory inhalation.
    B. parenteral injection.
    C. topical absorption.
    D. gastrointestinal ingestion.
    E. both A and C.

14. In a hazmat situation, the most common route(s) of exposure is (are) through
    A. respiratory inhalation.
    B. parenteral injection.
    C. topical absorption.
    D. gastrointestinal ingestion.
    E. both B and D.

15. If a patient was exposed to a hazardous gas and developed acute bronchospasm, this could be called a _____ effect.
    A. local
    B. systemic
    C. biotransformation
    D. synergistic
    E. secondary

16. The most common route of exposure of cyanides is through inhalation, although cyanides can also be ingested, absorbed, or injected.
    A. True
    B. False

17. Definitive treatment for CO inhalation is
    A. oxygenation.
    B. hyperbaric therapy.
    C. use of a cyanide kit.
    D. infusion of sodium thiosulfate.
    E. none of the above.

18. All of the following are methods of decontamination, EXCEPT
    A. stabilization.
    B. dilution.
    C. absorption.
    D. isolation.
    E. neutralization.

©2013 Pearson Education, Inc.
*Paramedic Care: Principles & Practice, Vol. 7, 4th Ed.*

_____ 19. Which priority should guide your decision making while performing decontamination?
- **A.** Life safety
- **B.** Incident stabilization
- **C.** Property conservation
- **D.** Triage
- **E.** Neutralization

_____ 20. All the following are common decontamination solvents, EXCEPT
- **A.** water.
- **B.** tincture of green soap.
- **C.** isopropyl alcohol.
- **D.** baking soda.
- **E.** vegetable oil.

_____ 21. Two methods for decontamination in the field are the
- **A.** two-step and twelve-step processes.
- **B.** complete and incomplete methods.
- **C.** gross decon and neutralizing methods.
- **D.** two-step and eight-step processes.
- **E.** fast-break and long-term methods.

_____ 22. The lowest level of hazmat protective equipment is
- **A.** Level A.
- **B.** Level B.
- **C.** Level C.
- **D.** Level D.
- **E.** Level E.

_____ 23. The highest level of hazmat protective equipment uses a(n)
- **A.** HEPA filter mask.
- **B.** air-purifying respirator.
- **C.** SCBA.
- **D.** SCUBA.
- **E.** PBI flash protector.

_____ 24. One of the primary roles of EMS personnel at a hazmat incident is medical monitoring of entry personnel.
- **A.** True
- **B.** False

_____ 25. Which of the following should be included in pre-entry and post-exit documentation?
- **A.** Body weight
- **B.** Pulse, respirations, and blood pressure
- **C.** ECG and temperature
- **D.** Mental/neurologic status
- **E.** All of the above

# MATCHING

_Write the letter of the term in the space provided next to the appropriate description._

- **A.** boiling point
- **B.** warm zone
- **C.** CHEMTREC
- **D.** hazardous material
- **E.** flash point
- **F.** ignition temperature
- **G.** cold zone
- **H.** warning placard
- **I.** MSDS
- **J.** hot zone

_____ 26. Any substance that causes adverse health effects upon human exposure

_____ 27. Diamond-shaped graphic placed on vehicles to indicate hazmat classification

_____ 28. Easily accessible sheets of detailed information about chemicals found at fixed facilities

_____ **29.** Chemical Transportation Emergency Center, which maintains a 24-hour toll-free hazmat information hotline

_____ **30.** The location where the hazardous material and the highest levels of contamination exist

_____ **31.** The location where the decontamination corridor should be set up

_____ **32.** The area at a hazardous materials incident where the command post and sectors are set up

_____ **33.** The lowest temperature at which a liquid will give off enough vapors to ignite

_____ **34.** The temperature at which a liquid becomes a gas

_____ **35.** The lowest temperature at which a liquid will give off enough vapors to support combustion

# Special Project

*Awareness Level Practice*

To participate effectively in a hazmat incident, you need to be familiar with the regulations and standards that guide operations during these emergencies. You will also need to know how to identify the hazardous substances involved at the incident. To be a more valuable and informed member of a hazmat emergency operation, complete these activities.

## Part I: Regulations and Standards

*Obtain a copy of the following regulations and review them to determine how they apply to you and your agency. Record information in the spaces provided.*

**OSHA CFR 1910.120**

Main Provisions: _____

_____

Local Application: _____

_____

_____

_____

**EPA 40 CFR 311**

Main Provisions: _____     _____

_____

Local Application: _____

_____

_____

_____

**NFPA 473**

Main Provisions: _____

Local Application: _____

_____

_____

_____

©2013 Pearson Education, Inc.
*Paramedic Care: Principles & Practice, Vol. 7, 4th Ed.*

## Part II: Identifying Hazardous Substances

*Obtain the latest copy of the Emergency Response Guidebook (ERG). After reviewing the book's format, find an example of a chemical in each of the following UN classifications. Write down the name of the substance and any special precautions that should be taken when you find this substance at a hazmat incident.*

| UN Classification | Chemical Name | Special Precautions to Take |
|---|---|---|
| 1 | | |
| 2 | | |
| 3 | | |
| 4 | | |
| 5 | | |
| 6 | | |
| 7 | | |
| 8 | | |
| 9 | | |

# 6

# Crime Scene Awareness

## Review of Chapter Objectives

### After reading this chapter, you should be able to:

1. **Define key terms introduced in this chapter.** **p. 112**

   Knowing and being able to apply the key terms in each chapter is critical to understanding chapter concepts. Write the list of key terms. Then write the definition of each one in your own words. Check your understanding by confirming the definitions in the text glossary. Correct any misunderstandings. Create a study aid by writing each key term on the front of an index card and the definition on the back. Use the cards to quiz yourself, or to have someone quiz you.

2. **Describe the demographics of violence.** **p. 113**

   Violence can occur anywhere. Regardless of where you work as a paramedic—the inner city, the suburbs, or rural America—you can be affected by violence. The violence can take all forms, from interpersonal abuse in the home to gang activities on the street. The violence can also involve any number of weapons, ranging from fists to guns to explosives.

   According to the Division of Violence Prevention at the National Center for Injury Prevention and Control, arrest rates for homicide, rape, robbery, and aggravated assault are consistently higher for people ages 15 to 34 than for all other age groups. Even more alarming, an average of 16 youth (ages 10–24) homicides occur in the United States every day. Among 10- to 24-year-olds, homicide is the leading cause of death for African Americans and the second leading cause of death for Hispanics. Approximately one of six victims of violent crimes requires medical attention, often by the emergency medical services.

   A more recent phenomenon is bullying. Bullying is a form of youth violence and can result in physical injury, social and emotional distress, and even death. Victimized youth are at increased risk for mental health problems such as depression and anxiety, psychosomatic complaints such as headaches, and poor school adjustment. Youth who bully others are at increased risk for substance use, academic problems, and violence later in adolescence and adulthood.

3. **Recognize indications that you may encounter violence on a call.** **p. 114**

   Your safety strategy begins as soon as you are dispatched on a call. Even the most basic information can provide important tactical clues. Emergency medical dispatchers try to keep callers on the line to obtain as much information as possible. They remain alert to background noises such as fighting or intoxicated persons, so they can warn incoming units of these dangers.

   Modern computer-aided dispatch programs provide instant information on previous calls at a particular location and display "caution indicators" to notify dispatchers when a location has a history of violence.

Even in the age of computers, however, some of your best information can still come from your own experience and that of other crews. Your memory of previous calls can serve as an important indicator of trouble.

One of the main purposes of the scene size-up is to search for any possible hazards. Even if dispatch has not alerted you to danger, you must still keep this possibility in mind once you arrive on the scene. Listen and observe for signs of danger. If you can, look in windows for evidence of fighting, the presence of weapons, or the use of alcohol or drugs. Listen for any signs of danger, such as loud noises, items breaking, incoherent speech, or the lack of any sounds at all. Remain alert throughout a call, especially in areas with a history of violence.

4. **Describe the actions you should take to protect your safety when you are advised of danger before you reach the scene, observe danger upon arriving at the scene, and when danger arises during a call.**    pp. 114–116

When the dispatcher reports possible danger, do not approach the scene until it has been secured by law enforcement personnel. Remember that lights and sirens can draw a crowd and/or alert the perpetrator of a crime, so use them cautiously or not at all.

Never follow police units to the scene. To do so might place you at the center of violence. If you arrive first, keep the ambulance out of sight so that the rig does not attract the attention of bystanders or any of the parties involved in the incident. While you wait for police to secure the scene, set up a staging area. Communicate with the police. Work with police to determine if and when you should approach the scene.

Keep in mind that violence can occur or resume even with the police present. Furthermore, depending on your uniform colors and the use of badges, people might mistake you for the police, especially if you exit from a vehicle with flashing lights and siren. They might expect you to intervene in a violent situation, or they might direct aggression toward you as an authority figure. If the scene cannot be made safe, retreat immediately.

Even if dispatch has not alerted you to danger, you must still keep this possibility in mind once you arrive on the scene. One of the main purposes of the scene size-up is to search for any possible hazards. This includes nonviolent dangers such as downed power lines, dangerous pets, unstable vehicles, or hazmat. As you look for these dangers, observe for other signs of trouble, such as crowds gathering on the street, an unusual silence, or a darkened residence. Obviously, you will adopt a different approach for a confirmed medical emergency than for an "unknown problem, caller hang-up." Even so, do not exit the vehicle until you have ruled out all immediate hazards.

If you have any doubts about a call, park away from the scene. If you must park in view of the location, take an unconventional approach to the door. People will expect you to use the sidewalk. So approach from the side, on the lawn, or flush against the house. Avoid getting between a residence and the lighted ambulance so you do not "backlight" yourself. Also, hold your flashlight to the side rather than in front of you. Armed assailants often fire at the light.

Before announcing your presence, listen and observe for signs of danger. If you can, look in windows for evidence of fighting, the presence of weapons, or the use of alcohol or drugs. Gradually make your way to the doorknob side of the door, or the side of the door opposite the hinges. Listen for any signs of danger such as loud noises, items breaking, incoherent speech, or the lack of any sounds at all.

If you spot danger at any time during your approach, immediately stop and reevaluate the situation. Decide whether it is in the interest of your own safety to continue or to retreat until law enforcement officials can be summoned. Rather than risk becoming injured or killed, err on the side of safety.

Remain alert throughout a call, especially in areas with a history of violence. You may enter the scene and spot weapons or drugs. Additional combative people may arrive on scene. The patient or bystanders may become agitated or threatening. Even if treatment has begun, you must place your own safety first. You now have two tactical options: (1) quickly package the patient and leave the scene with the patient or (2) retreat without the patient.

Your choice of action depends on the level of danger. Abandonment is always a concern. However, in most cases, you can legally leave a patient behind when there is a documented danger. Keep accurate records of incidents involving violence. If you must defend yourself, use the minimum amount of force necessary. Immediately summon police and retreat as needed.

©2013 Pearson Education, Inc.
*Paramedic Care: Principles & Practice, Vol. 7, 4th Ed.*

Regardless of the situation, always have a way out. Your failure to plan will undoubtedly lead to an emergency at some point in time. Make sure that standard operating procedures (SOPs) include an escape plan. Then adhere to this plan so you do not become a victim of violence yourself.

**5. Take steps to avoid the types of dangers you may encounter when responding to calls on the roadside or highway.** p. 116

EMS units frequently report to roadside calls involving motor vehicle collisions, disabled vehicles, or sick and/or unresponsive people inside a car, for example, "man slumped over wheel" calls. Highway operations also hold the risk of violence from occupants who may be intoxicated or drugged, fleeing from the police, or in possession of weapons. Some potential warning signs of danger include violent or abusive behavior, an altered mental state, grabbing or hiding items inside the vehicle, arguing or fighting among passengers, lack of activity where activity is expected, physical signs of alcohol or drug abuse, open or unlatched trunks, and differences among stories told by occupants.

To make a safe approach to a vehicle at a roadside emergency, follow these steps:

- Park the ambulance in a position that provides safety from traffic.
- Notify dispatch of the situation, location, the vehicle make and model, and the state and number of the license plate.
- Use a one-person approach. The driver should remain in the ambulance, which is elevated and provides greater visibility.
- The driver should remain prepared to radio for immediate help and to back or drive away rapidly once the other medic returns.
- At nighttime, use the ambulance lights to illuminate the vehicle. However, do not walk between the ambulance and the other vehicle. You will be backlighted, forming an easy target.
- Because police approach vehicles from the driver's side, you should approach from the passenger's side—an unexpected route.
- Use the A, B, and C door posts for cover.
- Observe the rear seat. Do not move forward of the C post unless you are sure there are no threats in the rear seat or foot wells.
- Retreat to the ambulance (or another strategic position of cover) at the first sign of danger.
- Make sure you have mapped out your intended retreat and escape with the ambulance driver.

**6. Take steps to avoid the types of dangers you may encounter when responding to violent street events.** pp. 116–118

You can encounter many different types of violence while working on the streets. Incidents can range from random acts of violence against individual citizens to organized efforts at domestic or international terrorism.

**Murder, Assault, and Robbery.** According to the U.S. Department of Justice, the most common location for violent crimes is on the streets. In order of occurrence, the most frequent crimes include simple assaults, aggravated assaults, rapes and sexual assaults, robberies, and homicides. The late 1990s and early 2000s saw a rise in hate crimes—crimes committed against a person solely on the basis of the individual's actual or perceived race, color, national origin, ethnicity, gender, disability, or sexual orientation.

In responding to the scene of any violent crime, keep these precautions in mind: dangerous weapons may have been used in the crime, perpetrators may still be on scene or could return to the scene, and patients may sometimes exhibit violence toward EMS, particularly if they risk criminal penalties as a result of the original incident.

**Dangerous Crowds and Bystanders.** You must remain aware of crowd dynamics whenever you respond to a street incident. Crowds can quickly become large and volatile, especially in the case of a hate crime. Violence can be directed against anyone or anything in the path of an angry crowd. Your status as an EMS provider does not give you immunity against an out-of-control mob.

Whenever a crowd is present, look for these warning signs of impending danger: shouts or increasingly loud voices, pushing or shoving, hostilities toward anyone on the scene, rapid increase in crowd size, and inability of law enforcement officials to control bystanders.

To protect yourself, constantly monitor the crowd and retreat if necessary. If possible, take the patient with you so that you do not have to return later. Rapid transport may require limited or tactical assessment at the scene with more in-depth assessment done inside the safety of the ambulance. Be sure to document reasons for the quick assessment and transport.

**Street Gangs.** Gangs include groups of people who band together for a variety of reasons: fraternization, self-protection, creation of a surrogate family, or, most frequently, for the pursuit of criminal enterprises. Street gangs can be found in big cities, suburban towns, and lately in rural America. No EMS unit is totally immune from gang activity. In fact, some organized gangs have purposely branched out into smaller towns in an effort to escape surveillance and expand their illicit businesses.

In some places, gangs have used firebombs, Molotov cocktails, and, on a limited basis, military explosives (hand grenades) as weapons of revenge and intimidation. Links have been drawn between street gangs and the sale of drugs, which in turn finances gang activities. Commonly observed gang characteristics include: appearance, graffiti, tattoos, and hand signals/language.

EMS units venturing into gang territory must be extremely cautious because of the potential for violence. Danger is increased if your uniform looks similar to the uniform worn by police. Gangs with a history of arrest may in fact make every effort to prevent you from transporting one of their members to a hospital or any other place beyond the reach of the gang. Do not force the issue if your safety is at stake.

**Drug-Related Crimes.** The sale of drugs goes hand in hand with violence. Hundreds of people die each year in drug deals gone bad. In addition, drug dealers protect their drug stashes and "shooting galleries" with booby traps, weapons, and abused dogs that are likely to attack. The combination of a high cash flow, addiction, and automatic weapons threatens anyone who unwittingly walks onto the scene of a drug deal or threatens to uncover an illicit drug operation.

A number of signs can alert you to the involvement of drugs at an EMS call: prior history of drugs in the neighborhood of the call, clinical evidence that the patient has used drugs of some kind, drug-related comments by bystanders, drug paraphernalia visible at the scene, and chemical odors or residues.

Whenever you observe any of the preceding items, assume the use or presence of drugs at the scene. Even if the patient is not involved, others at the scene may still pose a danger. Keep in mind that not all patients who use drugs will be seeking to harm you. Some may, in fact, be looking for help. Evaluate each situation carefully. Above all else, remember to retreat and/or request police backup at the earliest sign of danger.

7. **Describe particular safety concerns related to responding to clandestine drug laboratories.** pp. 118–119

Drug raids on clan labs have a way of turning into hazmat operations. All too often, the labs contain toxic fumes and volatile chemicals. The people on the scene complicate matters by fighting or shooting at the rescuers who come to extricate them from the toxic environment. As they retreat, drug dealers may also trigger booby traps or wait for police or EMS personnel to trigger them. If you ever come upon a clan lab, take these actions:

- Leave the area immediately
- Do not touch anything
- Never stop any chemical reactions already in progress
- Do not smoke or bring any source of flame near the lab
- Notify the police
- Initiate IMS and hazmat procedures
- Consider evacuation of the area

Remember that laboratories can be found anywhere—on farms, in trailers, in city apartments, and elsewhere. They may be mobile, roaming from place to place in a camper or truck. Or they may be disassembled and stored in almost any variety of locations. The job of raiding clan labs belongs to specialized personnel—not EMS crews.

©2013 Pearson Education, Inc.
*Paramedic Care: Principles & Practice, Vol. 7, 4th Ed.*

**8. Implement the tactical options of retreat, concealment, cover, distraction, evasion, contact and cover, warning signals, and communication when situations call for their use.**                                                   pp. 119–121

Your response to dangerous situations will be most effective if you practice tactical options frequently. Even on routine calls, think about safety, contact and cover, escape routes, and other strategies that can help you make a better decision when you are faced with actual danger. If you have rehearsed the responses to danger before you actually need them, you will be more likely to use them successfully.

**Retreat.** The prudent strategy is to retreat whenever you spot indicators of violence or potential physical confrontations, particularly with fleeing criminals or people with emotional disturbance. Retreat in a calm but decisive manner. Be aware that the danger is now at your back and integrate cover into your retreat.

Ideally, you will retreat to the ambulance so that you can summon help. However, if a dangerous obstacle, such as a crowd, blocks access to your rig, retreat by foot or by whatever means possible. Nothing in the ambulance is worth your life.

In deciding how far to retreat, your primary goal is to protect yourself from any potential danger. You must be out of the immediate line of sight. You must also seek cover from gunfire. Finally, you must allow enough distance to react if a person or crowd attempts to move toward you again. You need time and space to respond to changing situations.

As soon as possible, notify other responding units and agencies of the danger. Activate appropriate codes, SOPs, and/or interagency agreements, particularly with law enforcement departments. Be sure to document your observations of danger and your specific responses. Include information such as: actions taken while on the scene, reasons you retreated, time at which you left and/or returned to the scene, and personnel or agencies contacted.

Also keep in mind that retreat does not mean the end of a call. As already mentioned, you should seek to stage at a safe area until police secure the scene and you can respond once again. Staging, along with thorough documentation, will reduce liability and provide evidence to refute charges of abandonment.

**Cover and Concealment.** When faced with danger, two of your most immediate and practical strategies are cover and concealment. Concealment hides your body, such as when you crouch behind bushes, wallboards, or vehicle doors. During armed encounters, seek cover by hiding your body behind solid and impenetrable objects such as brick walls, rocks, large trees or telephone poles, and the engine block of vehicles.

As you approach any scene, remain aware of the surroundings and any potential sources of protection in case you must retreat or are "pinned down." Choose your cover carefully. You may have only one chance to pick your protection. Select the item that hides your body adequately, while shielding you against ballistics. Once you have made your choice of cover, conceal as much of your body as possible. Be conscious of any reflective clothing that you may be wearing. Armed assailants can use it as a target, especially at night. Constantly look to improve your protection and location.

**Distraction and Evasion.** Distraction and evasion can be integrated into any retreat. Some specific techniques to avoid physical violence include: throwing equipment to trip, slow, or distract an aggressor; wedging a stretcher in a doorway to block an attacker; using an unconventional path while retreating; anticipating the moves of the aggressor and taking countermoves; overturning objects in the path of the attacker; and using preplanned tactics with your partner to confuse or "throw off" an aggressor.

The key to the success of these safety tactics is your own physical well-being. Regular exercise and good health ensure that you will have the strength to outrun or, if necessary, defend yourself against an attacker. Some units provide basic training in self-defense or have protocols on its use. Make sure you take advantage of this training and/or know the protocols related to the application of force.

**Contact and Cover.** The San Diego Police Department adopted an interview approach in which one officer "contacts" the suspect while another officer stands 90 degrees to the side. By standing at a different angle, the second officer can provide "cover" to the officer dealing with the suspect.

As with any tactic adopted from another discipline, contact and cover has obvious correlations and drawbacks. The tactic is ideal for street encounters with intoxicated persons or subjects acting in a suspicious manner. An obvious drawback is that two medics working on a cardiac arrest will not be able to designate one person to act solely as a "cover" medic.

Perhaps the best application of this police procedure to EMS is its emphasis on the importance of observation and teamwork. A crew that works well together will assign roles—formally or informally—to guarantee safety and patient care. In its most basic form, contact and cover means that you will watch your partner's back while he watches yours.

**Warning Signals and Communication.** Communication forms a vital part of EMS, regardless of the situation. In the case of "street survival," it is an invaluable safety tool. Every team or crew should develop methods of alerting other providers to danger without alerting the aggressor. Devise prearranged verbal and nonverbal clues and then practice them.

Be sure to involve dispatch in the process. Choose signals that will indicate a variety of circumstances while sounding harmless to an attacker. This can be a lifesaving technique in situations where you find yourself, the crew, and/or the patient held hostage. Your so-called "routine" radio reports can spell out the nature of the trouble and summon help.

9. **Describe the advantages and limitations of using body armor.**                    p. 121

Unlike conventional armor, body armor is soft. A series of fibers such as Kevlar™ is woven tightly together to form the vest. The tight weave and strength of the material offer protection from many handgun bullets, most knives, and blunt trauma. The number of layers of fiber determine the rating or "stopping power" of a vest.

Some critics of body armor claim that wearers may feel a false sense of security. They point out that body armor offers reduced protection when wet. They also note that it provides little or no protection against high-velocity bullets, such as those fired by a rifle, or from thin or dual-edged weapons. An ice pick, for example, can penetrate between the fibers of most vests.

Supporters of body armor feel that it should be viewed just like any other personal protective equipment (PPE) offered to rescuers. They point to the new threats faced by emergency responders, such as paramilitary groups, international terrorists, drug-related violence, and the widespread possession of handguns.

Never do anything wearing body armor you wouldn't do without it. Remember that body armor doesn't cover the whole body. You can still get seriously injured or killed. Even though body armor can prevent many types of penetration, you can still experience severe cavitation. For body armor to work, it must be worn. The temptation not to wear it, especially in hot temperatures, can render even the best body armor useless.

10. **Describe the role of tactical EMS.**                    pp. 121–122

Tactical EMS (TEMS) requires special training and authorization. Like hazmat teams, they must don special equipment, function with compact gear, and, in most cases, work as medical adjuncts to the police or military.

The patient care offered by TEMS differs from routine EMS care in several ways:

- A major priority is extraction of the patient from the hot zone
- Care may be modified to meet tactical considerations
- Trauma patients are more frequently encountered than medical patients
- Treatment and transport interventions must almost always be coordinated with an incident commander
- Patients must be moved to tactically cold zones for complete assessment, care, and transport
- Metal clipboards, chemical agents, and other tools may be used as defensive weapons

The units may be composed of EMTs, paramedics, and/or physicians who operate as part of a tactical law enforcement team. The training required of EMT-Tacticals (EMT-Ts) or SWAT-Medics involves strenuous physical activity, under a variety of conditions. In a Counter-Narcotics Tactical Operations (CONTOMS) program, medics may be exposed to a variety of scenarios and skills.

©2013 Pearson Education, Inc.
*Paramedic Care: Principles & Practice, Vol. 7, 4th Ed.*

11. **Given a crime scene scenario, interact cooperatively with law enforcement to provide patient care while maintaining awareness of crime scene and evidence considerations.** pp. 122–124

Often emergencies arise where police and EMS personnel respond to the same crisis. Both are there for specific purposes. The EMS crew has arrived on the scene to treat patients and save lives. Law enforcement officers have come to protect the public and to solve a crime. These two primary goals sometimes create tension between the two teams.

The key to cooperation between EMS and law enforcement personnel is communication. You should become aware of the nature and significance of physical evidence at a crime scene and, if possible, keep that evidence intact. Police, on the other hand, should be aware that the first and foremost responsibility of a paramedic is to save the life of the victim. EMS personnel and law enforcement are really on the same side. Talk to each other.

Be aware that anything on and around the patient may be evidence. You never know when a seemingly unimportant item may in fact be crucial evidence that could help solve a crime. Whenever in doubt, save or treat an object as evidence.

Although the paramedic's primary responsibilities are scene safety and care of the patient, it is important to be cognizant of crime scene evidence and make every effort to avoid contaminating or disturbing it.

Gathering evidence is a specialized and time-consuming job. Although it is unrealistic to train EMS personnel in the details of police work, it is not unrealistic to ask them to develop an awareness of the general types of evidence that they may expect to encounter at a crime scene. Some of the main categories of evidence include prints, blood and body fluids, particulate evidence, and your own observations at the scene.

As a paramedic, you have two concerns when it comes to fingerprints. First, try not to disturb any fingerprint evidence that may be present. Second, do not leave behind your own fingerprints at a crime scene. Because of Standard Precautions, you will be wearing disposable gloves as a part of infection control. These gloves prevent you from leaving your own fingerprints. But they will not prevent you from smudging existing prints. Again, touch as little as possible. Also, bring in only the necessary equipment. The more equipment you have, the more evidence you can potentially disturb, including fingerprints.

The way in which blood is splattered or dropped at the scene provides yet other clues for police. This so-called blood spatter evidence can indicate the type of weapon used, the position of the attacker in relation to the victim, and the direction or force used in the attack. Preserving blood evidence can be performed in the following ways:

- Avoid mixing samples of blood whenever possible
- Avoid tracking blood on your shoes
- If you must cut bloody clothing from a victim, place each piece in a separate brown paper bag
- Do not throw clothes stained with blood or other body fluids in a single pile or in a puddle of blood
- Do not clean up or smudge blood spatter left at a scene
- If you leave behind blood from a venipuncture, notify police
- Because blood can be a biohazard, ask police whether the scene should be secured for evidence collection

Particulate evidence can help identify the actual crime scene, such as in cases where a body has been moved, or the DNA of the perpetrator. Minimal handling of a victim's clothes by EMS personnel may help to preserve this evidence.

Everything that you and other members of the EMS crew see and hear can serve as evidence. Your observations of the scene will become part of the police record—and ultimately part of the court record. Be sure to look for and record the following information:

- Conditions at the scene (e.g., absence or presence of lights, locked or unlocked doors, open or closed curtains)
- Position of the patient/victim
- Injuries suffered by the patient/victim
- Statements of persons at the scene
- Statements by the patient/victim

- Dying declarations
- Suspicious persons at, or fleeing from, the scene
- Presence and/or location of any weapons

If the victim is deceased by the time you arrive, any staff not immediately needed on the scene should leave to minimize the risk of disturbing evidence.

Record only the facts at the scene of a crime, and record them accurately. Use quotation marks to indicate the words of bystanders and any remarks made by the patient. Avoid opinions not relevant to patient care. If the patient has died, do not offer any judgments that might contradict later findings by the medical examiner. Also keep in mind the protocols, local laws, and ethical considerations in reporting certain crimes, such as child abuse, rape, geriatric abuse, and domestic violence. Finally, follow local policies and regulations regarding confidentiality surrounding any criminal case. Any offhand remarks that you make might later become testimony in a courtroom along with other documents that you prepare at the scene.

# Case Study Review

*Reread the case study on page 113 in* Paramedic Care: Operations; *then, read the following discussion.*

*This case underscores the cautious approach that should be used with any scene that holds the potential for violence. Although this turned out to be a routine call, the paramedics had no way of knowing that during the initial phases of the incident.*

A quiet call can be just as dangerous as a call that involves shouting, yelling, and other obvious signs of potential violence. You should not drop your guard just because the call is in a "well-kept" neighborhood or the patient is "too old" or "too young" to be capable of violence. In this case, the paramedics park the ambulance a safe distance from the house and observe through the windshield before exiting the vehicle. They approach with only the necessary equipment, taking separate and unpredictable paths. After looking in the window, the paramedics deem the scene safe and approach the patient.

Even on routine runs, think about safety, contact and cover, escape routes, and other strategies that can help you make better decisions when you are faced with actual danger. Borrowing a phrase from professional sports: "You will play the game the way you practice." If you have rehearsed the responses to danger before you actually need them, you will be more likely to use them successfully.

# Content Self-Evaluation

## MULTIPLE CHOICE

_____ 1. According to the Division of Violence Prevention at the National Center for Injury Prevention, arrest rates for homicide, rape, robbery, and aggravated assault are consistently higher for people ages
A. 10 to 14.
B. 15 to 34.
C. 35 to 50.
D. 51 to 65.
E. over 65.

_____ 2. A computer-aided dispatch (CAD) program can assist in preventing an attack on EMS personnel by
A. predicting when crimes are most likely to occur.
B. noting addresses with a history of violence.
C. maintaining a list of known criminals.
D. linking an EMS unit to a special forces team.
E. all of the above.

©2013 Pearson Education, Inc.
*Paramedic Care: Principles & Practice, Vol. 7, 4th Ed.*

_____ 3. The EMS unit should follow the police units to the scene.
   A. True
   B. False

_____ 4. One of the main purposes of the scene size-up at a crime scene is to search for
   A. possible evidence.
   B. alleged assailants.
   C. hazards.
   D. law enforcement officials.
   E. a way to rescue the victim.

_____ 5. Even if a scene has been declared secure by the police, violence may still occur.
   A. True
   B. False

_____ 6. When approaching a residence that may be hazardous, you should
   A. be careful not to backlight yourself.
   B. hold your flashlight to the side.
   C. take an unconventional approach to the door.
   D. keep your partner in sight.
   E. all of the above.

_____ 7. Before knocking on the door, you should do all of the following, EXCEPT
   A. stand on the hinge side of the door.
   B. listen for loud noises.
   C. listen for items breaking.
   D. listen for the lack of any sounds at all.
   E. look in the windows for the presence of weapons.

_____ 8. If you must defend yourself, use the maximum amount of force possible.
   A. True
   B. False

_____ 9. To make a safe approach to a suspicious roadside emergency, you should take all of the following safety steps, EXCEPT
   A. use a one-person approach.
   B. use the ambulance lights to illuminate the vehicle.
   C. approach the vehicle from the driver's side.
   D. use the A, B, and C posts for cover.
   E. observe the rear seat.

_____ 10. According to the U.S. Department of Justice, the most common location for violent crimes is on the streets.
   A. True
   B. False

_____ 11. Crimes committed against a person solely on the basis of the individual's actual or perceived race, color, national origin, ethnicity, gender, disability, or sexual orientation are known as
   A. bias crimes.
   B. hate crimes.
   C. nondiscriminatory crimes.
   D. selective crimes.
   E. none of the above.

_____ 12. When responding to the scene of any violent crime, you should remember that
   A. dangerous weapons may have been used in the crime.
   B. perpetrators may still be on the scene.
   C. patients may sometimes exhibit violence toward EMS personnel.
   D. perpetrators may return to the scene.
   E. all of the above.

_____ 13. Warning signs of impending danger from a crowd include all of the following, EXCEPT
   A. a rapid increase in crowd size.
   B. hostility toward anyone on the scene.
   C. pushing or shoving.
   D. inability of police to control bystanders.
   E. a decreasing level of noise.

_____ 14. Gang activities are confined to urban areas and are of minimal concern to EMS units outside cities.
   A. True
   B. False

_____ 15. A gang's "colors" refers to its
   A. clothing.
   B. flag.
   C. language.
   D. graffiti.
   E. logo.

_____ 16. One of the most common substances manufactured in clandestine drug labs is
   A. cocaine.
   B. methamphetamine.
   C. heroin.
   D. methadone.
   E. morphine.

_____ 17. Clan labs generally have the following requirements
   A. privacy.
   B. utilities.
   C. glassware.
   D. heating mantles or burners.
   E. all of the above.

_____ 18. If you ever come upon a clan lab, all of the following are appropriate actions, EXCEPT to
   A. leave the area immediately.
   B. stop any chemical reactions in progress.
   C. notify the police.
   D. initiate Incident Command System (ICS) and hazmat procedures.
   E. evacuate the area.

_____ 19. All of the following strategies can be employed as safety tactics in a potentially violent situation, EXCEPT
   A. retreat.
   B. cover and concealment.
   C. confrontation and interrogation.
   D. distraction and evasion.
   E. contact and cover.

_____ 20. Concealment is hiding your body behind solid and impenetrable objects such as brick walls.
   A. True
   B. False

_____ 21. Most body armor is able to stop all bullets and all but a few knives.
   A. True
   B. False

_____ 22. Which of the following describes how tactical EMS differs from normal or nontactical EMS?
   A. A major priority is patient extraction.
   B. Trauma is more frequent than medical emergencies.
   C. Treatment interventions must be coordinated with the incident commander (IC).
   D. Complete assessment occurs after patient movement.
   E. All of the above are differences between tactical and nontactical EMS.

_____ 23. Which of the following is NOT appropriate when providing care at the possible crime scene?
   A. Cut through bullet or knife holes in clothing.
   B. Place clothing in paper bags.
   C. Place patient care before crime scene preservation.
   D. Wear gloves and otherwise limit any fingerprints you might leave behind.
   E. All of the above are appropriate actions at a crime scene.

_____ 24. Gloves worn by EMS providers generally limit the fingerprints left behind at the scene but will not prevent other prints from being smudged.
   A. True
   B. False

©2013 Pearson Education, Inc.
_Paramedic Care: Principles & Practice, Vol. 7, 4th Ed._

_____ **25.** Which of the following is proper for documenting a crime scene response?

    **A.** Record only the facts at the crime scene.

    **B.** Use quotation marks to indicate exact words from bystanders or the patient.

    **C.** Do not offer opinions as to the victim's cause of death.

    **D.** Describe the nature and shape of a wound, not the suspected cause.

    **E.** All of the above are proper in documenting a crime scene response.

## MATCHING

*Write the letter of the term in the space provided next to the appropriate description.*

**A.** TEMS

**B.** particulate evidence

**C.** concealment

**D.** SWAT

**E.** body armor

**F.** EMT-Ts

**G.** blood splatter evidence

**H.** cover

**I.** CONTOMS

**J.** hate crimes

_____ **26.** Committed against a person solely on the basis of the individual's actual or perceived race, color, national origin, ethnicity, gender, disability, or sexual orientation

_____ **27.** Trained police unit equipped to handle hostage takers and other difficult law enforcement situations

_____ **28.** Hiding the body behind objects that shield a person from view but offer little or no protection against bullets or other ballistics

_____ **29.** Vest made of tightly woven, strong fibers that offers protection against handgun bullets, most knives, and blunt trauma

_____ **30.** Counter-narcotics tactical operations program that manages training and certification of EMT-Ts and SWAT-Medics

_____ **31.** Hairs or fibers that cannot be readily seen with the human eye

_____ **32.** A specially trained unit that provides on-site medical support to law enforcement

_____ **33.** Hiding the body behind solid and impenetrable objects that protect a person from bullets

_____ **34.** Pattern that blood forms when it is dropped at the scene of a crime

_____ **35.** EMS personnel trained to serve with a law enforcement agency

## SHORT ANSWER

### Part A

*List seven things that you or any member of an EMS team can do to preserve blood evidence at the scene of a crime*

**36.** _____

_____

37. _____

_____

38. _____

_____

39. _____

_____

40. _____

_____

41. _____

_____

42. _____

_____

## Part B

*In addition to blood and body fluids, list three other categories of evidence that EMS personnel should be aware of at a crime scene.*

43. _____

44. _____

45. _____

# Special Project

## Crime Hazard Awareness

*Take a walk around each room in your residence and inventory all the items that could easily be used as weapons against a responding paramedic. You should note things like ashtrays, scissors, letter openers, statues, and bottles—then there are all those knives in the woodblock on the kitchen counter!*

   *List the items you found:*

   **Living Room:** _____

_____

_____

   **Kitchen:** _____

_____

_____

   **Dining Room:** _____

_____

_____

   **Bedroom:** _____

_____

_____

©2013 Pearson Education, Inc.
*Paramedic Care: Principles & Practice, Vol. 7, 4th Ed.*

**Bathroom:** _____

_____

_____

# 7

# **Rural EMS**

## Review of Chapter Objectives

### **After reading this chapter, you should be able to:**

1.  **Define key terms introduced in this chapter.**                                       **p. 126**

    Knowing and being able to apply the key terms in each chapter is critical to understanding chapter concepts. Write the list of key terms. Then write the definition of each one in your own words. Check your understanding by confirming the definitions in the text glossary. Correct any misunderstandings. Create a study aid by writing each key term on the front of an index card and the definition on the back. Use the cards to quiz yourself, or to have someone quiz you.

2.  **Describe the demographics, health status, and health access issues of rural populations.**                                       **p. 128**

    Recent U.S. Census data indicate that more than 53 million people in the United States live in rural areas. In fact, some states have rural populations of nearly 50 percent or more. In general, the U.S. government defines rural areas in terms of their sparse populations and distances from cities, towns, or villages.

    People choose to live in rural areas for a variety of reasons. Their families have always lived there. They work at occupations such as farming, ranching, or mining. They like the solitude, open space, or recreational activities found in rural areas. Regardless of the reason, most rural dwellers face a similar problem: lack of easy access to the health care facilities found in most urban and suburban areas.

    In the rural setting, resources such as full-service hospitals, fire departments, and EMS units are often as thinly distributed as the population. Specialty teams may be nonexistent. One of the challenges for rural EMS providers is to ensure that their patients receive the same high-quality care as people living elsewhere in the nation.

    Rural areas can also be characterized by their higher percentage of people over age 65 and their lower physician-to-patient ratios. One in five people in the United States lives in rural settings, but only about 1 in 10 doctors chooses to practice in these locations.

    It has been found that rural residents experience a disproportionate number of serious injuries and chronic health conditions. Because of the greater distances to health care facilities, rural residents suffer a higher level of mortality associated with trauma and medical emergencies. In many cases, an EMS unit may provide the definitive care. In meeting the challenge of practicing rural EMS, paramedics and other health care personnel need to be aware of the special problems facing them.

3.  **Describe the special problems faced by rural EMS systems.**                                       **pp. 128–130**

    Regardless of the circumstances surrounding a call, rural EMS crews face a number of obstacles and challenges not found in most urban areas. As a paramedic, you will assume an expanded leadership role in directing other EMS personnel on how best to handle or overcome the following special problems.

    **Distance and Time.** Rural EMS often relies on volunteer services. In responding to calls, volunteers must first travel varying distances to a squad building. Once aboard the ambulance, they then travel the distance to the patient and later the distance to the hospital. As a result, every decision that a paramedic makes in a rural setting needs to be made with the thought of distance in mind.

**Communication Difficulties.** In rural areas, poor or old communication equipment often hampers public access to EMS. A rural area, for example, may not have universal access to 911. Lack of 911 service will delay response time or, in many cases, lead people to turn telephone operators into dispatchers.

Rural EMS crews can also be hampered by inadequate communications. Antiquated "fire phones" or "crash bars" might notify them of an emergency call, but crew members may have no way of communicating with each other en route to the service vehicle. Crews may also lack information from dispatch until they arrive at the squad building or are on board the ambulance.

While traveling on the ambulance, rural EMS providers may experience dead spots where they cannot transmit. Frequencies can also be overloaded with static from highway departments and school buses. This impairs a medic's ability to communicate with other ambulance crews or with medical direction. As a result, rural paramedics must often think ahead, asking for orders in anticipation of medical conditions that might develop while traveling within a dead spot.

**Enrollment Shortages.** Because many rural EMS providers work on a volunteer basis, units or squads can experience enrollment shortages. Volunteers must respond to calls from their jobs or homes. The greater distances and time involved in many rural EMS calls can take volunteers from their work or families for lengthy periods. This situation can affect their ability to earn a living or to raise their children. As a result, they often serve for only short stretches or resign entirely.

**Training and Practice.** Access to training and continuing education is not readily available in many rural areas. In addition, the cost and amount of time required for certification as a paramedic has increased. For the volunteer, this means increased personal expense and time away from home. The net effect can be EMS providers with a less advanced level of training than their paid urban counterparts.

This situation can be further complicated by the low volume of EMS calls in some rural areas. EMS providers simply do not have the opportunity to practice their skills on a consistent basis. Members of rescue squads may experience what has become known as rust out, or an inability to keep abreast of new technologies and standards.

**Inadequate Medical Support.** As might be expected, rural areas sometimes have inadequate medical direction. Local physicians may lack the training in EMS operations or feel EMS operations should not be part of their job.

Rural areas also may not have the budgets to buy new equipment and ambulances. In addition, air medical transport may not always be readily available due to many factors, such as distance, lack of landing areas, cost, or too few helicopters for a large area.

Hospitals and rural EMS agencies may not always implement protocols or standards for prehospital providers. Roles may not be clearly defined, or hospitals may have varying protocols. A rural paramedic faced with the decision to transport a patient to two different hospitals may have to deal with two different sets of protocols for prehospital care. That means that volunteers must seek out and familiarize themselves with these protocols, often on their own.

4. **Suggest solutions to solving special problems faced by rural EMS systems.** pp. 130–131

**Improved Communications.** In recent years, some rural counties have been fortunate enough to receive grants to modernize or supplement their communications equipment. In other areas, rural counties have joined together to share in the cost of implementing 911 systems. As 911 systems enter rural areas, dispatchers gain valuable education in medical priority dispatch and medical-assist dispatch. Dispatchers with specialized training can provide lifesaving instructions while rural crews are en route to emergencies.

Radio dead spots and crowded frequencies can be handled by requesting additional frequencies and/or by upgrading radio equipment. One possible solution is more powerful base station radios and towers. A group effort in the form of a 911 user advisory board or consortium of agencies can help reduce or eliminate the problem of radio traffic overcrowding. Such advisory boards or consortiums can also provide a forum for discussion of common communication concerns and other issues.

©2013 Pearson Education, Inc.
*Paramedic Care: Principles & Practice, Vol. 7, 4th Ed.*

A technological innovation that promises to improve communications in rural areas is the cell phone. Through the use of cell phones, rural paramedics can communicate with emergency department physicians or their medical directors. Another innovation currently under consideration is the designation of cells for EMS use only.

**Recruitment and Certification.** Recognizing the problem of distance, units with paramedics on board can intercept basic life support (BLS) crews that require advanced life-support measures for their patients. Paramedic units can thus help ensure the highest level of service in rural counties.

The issues of recruitment and certification of paramedics in rural areas can be addressed through flexible training sessions and ongoing education.

To increase interest in volunteer EMS, rural agencies can utilize "explorer" and "ride-along" programs, when appropriate. Paramedics can serve as "recruiters" by taking the lead in training rural residents as cardiopulmonary resuscitation (CPR) drivers or first responders. The goal is to involve them in ambulance service or quick-response units as soon as possible. Once part of the EMS system, these volunteers can be encouraged to advance to the EMT and paramedic levels of training.

Some of the most important training advancements for rural areas have come through the use of computers and the Internet. EMS personnel can use "distance learning" to develop an awareness of new standards and procedures. The Internet also provides rural squads with a cost-effective way to interface with other agencies. Networking over the Internet can be an excellent way to promote creative problem solving or to share new ideas.

Even without benefit of the Internet, agencies or units can purchase interactive CD-ROMs and EMS computer simulation programs. These programs allow crew members to maintain a high level of knowledge and skills.

**Improved Medical Support.** The National Association of EMS Physicians provides numerous educational opportunities for physicians interested in learning more about the supervision and oversight of EMS operations. Conferences held by this organization offer courses in EMS medical direction.

Regardless of where a paramedic lives, positive relationships with a hospital depend on good communications. A medic should spend time at the hospitals that serve his district and, when possible, request to sit in on relevant in-service training sessions provided for the hospital staff.

**Ingenuity and Increased Responsibilities.** Rural EMS requires ingenuity. For most rural agencies, it is a constant struggle to retain members, supplement budgets, update equipment, provide quality education programs, and network with other health care facilities. As a rural paramedic, you will be involved in most, if not all, of these aspects of rural EMS.

As a rural paramedic, you can expect your role to grow as counties attempt to fill the "health care gap" between rural and urban areas. You may find yourself involved in hospital outreach programs such as prompt care facilities, or agencies that provide limited care and nonemergent medical treatment. In such cases, you may work under the direction of a physician or a physician's assistant (PA) and administer immunizations, wound care, and provide emergent transport as necessary.

Governments in some rural areas are also considering the involvement of paramedics in the public health system when not responding to emergency calls. Whatever the future may hold, you will be challenged as a rural paramedic to raise the standard of prehospital care offered to the rural residents who make up nearly one-quarter of the nation's population.

5. **Given a variety of scenarios, integrate the special challenges and considerations of rural EMS into patient care decision making.** pp. 131–132

In rural settings, it is often necessary to travel great distances. As a result, you may spend far more time with the patient on board the ambulance than at the scene itself. With this in mind, actions taken by a rural paramedic during transport can have a definitive impact on the patient's outcome. During transport, for example, you could treat a congestive heart failure (CHF) patient with nitrates, continuous positive airway pressure (CPAP), and an angiotensin-converting enzyme (ACE) inhibitor. By the time you reach the hospital, the patient may be completely out of crisis. For this reason, you must keep accurate and complete documentation during any lengthy transport.

Another factor to consider during transport is the availability of emergency staff at the local hospital. In most urban areas, hospitals stay active all night. They have full-time emergency departments with around-the-clock staffing able to handle complicated procedures 24 hours a day, 7 days a week.

Some rural hospitals, however, may only have a part-time emergency department with only one or two doctors on staff. In such cases, you may have to contact the hospital from the scene to arrange for the necessary personnel to be in the building when you arrive. You may also have to make a judgment call on whether or not to transport a critically injured patient to a more distant full-time trauma center. In the case of cardiac problems, the availability of fibrinolytic or percutaneous coronary intervention (PCI) might be the deciding factor.

In rural EMS, every decision depends on the situation. Because paramedics live in a world of advanced cardiac life support and trauma life support, you may have access to advanced equipment that is unavailable at your local hospital. A rural hospital under budget constraints, for example, may be unable to purchase equipment such as 12-lead electrocardiogram (ECG) monitors and similar technology. In such instances, you might decide with approval of medical direction to use your equipment at the local hospital or to transport the patient to a definitive treatment center at a more distant location.

In treating seriously ill or injured patients, keep in mind that you may see all phases of a patient's death before reaching a distant medical facility. Consider a motor vehicle collision patient with a serious head trauma. At first, your patient may be alert, conscious, and oriented. The patient then becomes agitated and aggressive. He may begin to have memory lapses and become more confused. You notice dilated pupils. If the transport is long enough, the patient will go into a decorticate posture, then a decerebrate posture. You face this situation knowing that there is little or nothing you can do to change the patient outcome because of the unavoidable transport time.

6. **Recognize the particular hazards and considerations involved in agricultural emergencies.** pp. 132–137

Emergencies related to farming or ranching can range from equipment-related injuries to pesticide poisoning to any number of medical problems exacerbated by agricultural labor. As in any emergency situation, you must place crew safety first. Interpret the situation described by the dispatcher and think of all the scenarios that could be connected with this situation. In agricultural emergencies, many possibilities for injury exist. Potential dangers include livestock, chemicals, fuel tanks, fumes in storage bins and silos, and heavy or outdated farm equipment.

In general, provide the same emergency medical care to patients involved in agricultural emergencies as you would to any other patient with similar injuries. In addition, because of unsanitary work conditions, sepsis and poisoning are very real possibilities.

**Farm Machinery.** If you live in an agricultural area, you must familiarize yourself with the range of equipment used on farms or ranches. Farm equipment can be very different from a car, in which a simple turn of the key shuts off the vehicle.

To prevent on-scene injuries, you need to make sure that farm equipment is both stable and locked down. Keep in mind that many types of farm equipment have fuel line shutoffs or power-kill switches. For this reason, it is important that you place personnel familiar with the equipment in charge of shutting off and locking down all machinery. Keep in mind this safety principle: lock-out/tag-out. After you shut off the equipment, you lock off the switch and place a tag on the switch stating why it is shut off. This prevents accidental retripping of switches.

The possibility for injury exists even after the equipment has been turned off. Engines fueled by gasoline, diesel, or propane hold the potential for explosion. Equipment that is not properly stabilized or chained can still roll or turn over.

When lifting equipment, the center of gravity can shift, increasing the pressure on the patient or causing injury to crew members.

**Hazardous Materials.** Hazardous materials can be found in many places on a farm or ranch. They exist in greenhouses, bins used to store pesticides, the equipment used to spray or dust crops, and the manure storage pits on large livestock facilities. For this reason, a self-contained breathing apparatus (SCBA) should be standard equipment on every rural EMS unit.

Be especially wary of rescues involving grain tanks and silos. Over time, grain and silage will ferment if stored long enough. During fermentation, crops release high levels of carbon dioxide ($CO_2$), silo gas, and methane. In rescues involving silos, you face the added risk of high angles, confined spaces, and the possibility of entombment under grain or silage. In such cases, determine whether any

©2013 Pearson Education, Inc.
*Paramedic Care: Principles & Practice, Vol. 7, 4th Ed.*

other agencies might be needed at the scene. Keep in mind the distance factor; don't arrive at the scene to find out you lack the correct apparatus or support for the call.

**Potential for Trauma.** Many farmers or ranchers work seven days a week, from sunrise to sunset. They endure extremes of heat, cold, and all kinds of weather conditions. They may spend a large part of the day in remote areas, far from telephones and help if injured.

The risk of serious agricultural accidents and injuries is increased by the equipment and machines routinely used by farmers. In some cases, farmers rely on old or outdated equipment because they cannot afford to replace it. They often wear little or no protective gear and may attempt to repair dangerous equipment themselves. All of these situations expose farm workers to equipment-related trauma. Depending on the type of machinery, the mechanism of injury could be crushing, twisting, tearing, penetrating, or a combination of mechanisms.

Equipment-related trauma is complicated by a number of factors related to agriculture. First, a wound may become contaminated by pesticides or manure. Second, a patient may easily become trapped or entangled under heavy equipment, making extrication both difficult and time consuming. Standard extrication devices that are used efficiently for automobiles may be unable to handle the weight of heavy farm equipment. In some cases, extrication equipment may be unavailable and crews will need to improvise using other farm equipment.

Lengthy extrications can worsen the patient's condition. You might use air bags or cribbing to relieve some of the equipment's weight. However, if extrication goes on too long, a patient may suffer from compartment syndrome. This occurs when circulation to a portion of the body is cut off. Over a period of time (usually hours), toxins develop in the blood, and when circulation is restored the patient goes into shock. This is a serious complication that can be fatal unless proper treatment is given in a timely manner.

Suspect many different mechanisms of injury in accidents involving agricultural equipment. Most farm machinery has spinning parts, such as fans, power takeoff (PTO) shafts, augers, pulleys, and wheels. These can cause sprains, strains, avulsions, fractures, and possible amputations. Common mechanisms of injury include wrap points, pinch points, shear points, and crush points.

**7. Anticipate injuries associated with various recreational activities.**   pp. 137–139

Depending on the season and the activity, the population in a rural community can swell dramatically as vacationers, sports enthusiasts, or "adventurer-seekers" arrive in an area. As a rural paramedic, you need to be familiar with the recreational or wilderness pursuits in your area.

If you live near a lake, local lifeguards can perform basic first aid and CPR, but they cannot abandon their beach patrol. Further treatment and transport falls to local EMS units. In such cases, a paramedic would need to be well versed in the procedures and skills related to water emergencies.

If you live in a wilderness or mountainous area, you might need to be aware of the accidents commonly encountered by hunters, backpackers, mountaineers, rock climbers, or mountain bikers. You might decide to take courses to receive certification in wilderness rescue. You might also practice rescues in extreme weather conditions. In wilderness rescues, distance and extrication time play an important part in your decisions.

A helicopter might seem the obvious choice of transport for wilderness rescues. However, you must take into account weather conditions, availability of suitable landing zones, and the time it will take a helicopter to arrive. In some instances, ground transport may be more efficient, even if it means carrying a patient out in a basket stretcher. In other instances, a helicopter might be able to provide a higher level of care, depending on regional and state protocols. Keep in mind that the helicopter has specific uses, tied to distance and level of care. Indiscriminate use of air transport can sometimes add dangerous minutes to patient treatment or even carry the risk of further patient injury.

# Case Study Review

*Reread the case study on pages 127 and 128 in* Paramedic Care: Operations; *then, read the following discussion.*

This case study shows how, due to the "distance factor," rural ALS teams often spend more time with patients than they would in an urban setting. In the sample scenario, the team performs lifesaving interventions that compensate for the lengthy transport to a hospital.

As in any situation, safety was the top priority for the paramedics who responded to this call. Prior to actually assessing the patient, the crew sized up the scene to rule out hazardous materials or "silo gas"—very real possibilities in an agricultural setting. Once they appraised scene safety, they approached the patient to begin assessment.

Throughout the case, the issue of time is dealt with: "5 minutes to assemble and get a volunteer squad en route to the farm," "1 minute to get a full-time paid agency off the floor," "the downtime is now 40 minutes," "total time of treatment prior to transport is 11 minutes," and the implied time in stating that the patient "is taken to a local hospital 33 miles away." As you can see, distance made it difficult for the crew to adhere to the guideline of the Golden Period. Also, they probably spent more time with the patient en route to the hospital than they did on the scene.

Anticipating the possibility of dead spots—and changing patient conditions during a lengthy transport—the paramedics request additional orders from medical direction according to ALS protocols. The actions taken by this ALS crew, working with the volunteer BLS team, made the difference between life and death.

# Content Self-Evaluation

## MULTIPLE CHOICE

_____ 1. According to recent U.S. Census data, the number of people who live in rural parts of the United States is about
   A. 36 million.
   B. 42 million.
   C. 48 million.
   D. 53 million.
   E. 76 million.

_____ 2. It has been found that rural residents experience a disproportionate number of
   A. chronic health conditions.
   B. serious injuries.
   C. trauma-related mortalities.
   D. medical-related mortalities.
   E. all of the above.

_____ 3. In the case of natural disasters, rural EMS personnel may be the only available medical support.
   A. True
   B. False

_____ 4. All of the following complicate rural EMS, EXCEPT
   A. radio dead spots.
   B. use of cell phones.
   C. the distance factor.
   D. crowded frequencies.
   E. enrollment shortages.

_____ 5. One of the most important ways to improve rural EMS systems is the effort to increase the number of
   A. dispatchers.
   B. fire phones.
   C. paramedics.
   D. air medical helicopters.
   E. prompt care facilities.

©2013 Pearson Education, Inc.
*Paramedic Care: Principles & Practice, Vol. 7, 4th Ed.*

6. Rural paramedics must be highly skilled and highly practiced to compensate for the extended run times and more complicated logistics found in many rural settings.
   A. True
   B. False

7. What condition occurs when circulation to a portion of the body is cut off and toxins develop in the blood?
   A. Toxic-shock syndrome
   B. Compression syndrome
   C. Decompression syndrome
   D. Compartment syndrome
   E. None of the above

8. The risk of serious agricultural accidents and injuries is increased by
   A. the long distances to hospitals.
   B. equipment and machines routinely used by farmers.
   C. radio communications problems.
   D. lack of cooperation by rural patients.
   E. high percentage of people over 65.

9. All of the following are mechanisms of injury associated with agricultural equipment, EXCEPT
   A. wrap points.
   B. shear points.
   C. crush points.
   D. pinch points.
   E. push points.

10. In some instances, ground transport may be more efficient than air medical transport, even if it means carrying a patient out in a basket stretcher.
    A. True
    B. False

## MATCHING

*Write the letter of the term in the space provided next to the appropriate description.*

A. air bags

B. lock-out/tag-out

C. compartment syndrome

D. silo gas

E. rust out

F. wrap points

G. prompt care facilities

H. distance factor

I. cribbing

J. PTO

_____ 11. An inability to keep abreast of new technologies and standards

_____ 12. Hospital agencies that provide limited care and nonemergent medical treatment

_____ 13. Locking off of a machinery switch and then placing a tag on the switch stating why it is shut off

_____ 14. Fumes produced in a grain storage bin

_____ 15. Inflatable high-pressure pillows that, when inflated, can lift up to 20 tons, depending on the brand

_____ 16. Wooden slats used to shore up heavy equipment

_____ 17. Condition that occurs when circulation to a portion of the body is cut off

_____ 18. Mechanisms of injury in which an appendage gets caught and significantly twisted

_____ 19. Power takeoff

_____ 20. A consideration for the extended times to respond to, arrive at, and transport to a hospital facility

## SHORT ANSWER

*List five challenges faced in practicing EMS in rural areas.*

21. _____

22. _____

23. _____

24. _____

25. _____

# Special Project

## Going Online

*The Internet is an excellent resource that brings rural EMS agencies closer to urban and suburban services. Not only can you assess vital information from national EMS agencies, but you can also participate in continuing medical education.*

*Go online to find links to at least five sites that offer resources and information for rural EMS.*

Name of website: _____

URL: _____

Resources and information offered: _____

Name of website: _____

URL: _____

Resources and information offered: _____

Name of website: _____

URL: _____

Resources and information offered: _____

Name of website: _____

URL: _____

Resources and information offered: _____

Name of website: _____

URL: _____

Resources and information offered: _____

©2013 Pearson Education, Inc.
*Paramedic Care: Principles & Practice, Vol. 7, 4th Ed.*

# Responding to Terrorist Acts

## Review of Chapter Objectives

### After reading this chapter, you should be able to:

**1. Define key terms introduced in this chapter.**                          **pp. 141–142**

Knowing and being able to apply the key terms in each chapter is critical to understanding chapter concepts. Write the list of key terms. Then write the definition of each one in your own words. Check your understanding by confirming the definitions in the text glossary. Correct any misunderstandings. Create a study aid by writing each key term on the front of an index card and the definition on the back. Use the cards to quiz yourself, or to have someone quiz you.

**2. Identify likely targets of terrorist attacks.**                          **p. 143**

Terrorists may be of foreign or domestic origin. They are likely to target locations that are symbolic of the government (such as a federal building) or that represent the influence of a country (such as an embassy). Domestic terrorists may further target corporations or their executives who represent a threat to their cause. They may also target their own employer or the public through their employer's products. The objective of both the domestic and the foreign terrorist is to incite terror in the public.

**3. Identify information and observations that can indicate a potential terrorist attack when responding to calls.**                          **pp. 151–152**

It is relatively easy to recognize a nuclear or conventional explosion. However, remember that radioactive fallout travels with the upper wind currents (not just at ground level), so watch cloud movement. Remember, too, that terrorists may use the conventional explosion to distribute radioactive or other hazardous material (the "dirty bomb"), and they may set secondary detonations through booby traps or timers that are designed to target rescuers.

A chemical release may not be as obvious. There may or may not be a cloud of gas or aerosolized material. There also may or may not be any unusual odors. However, groups of victims will be complaining of similar symptoms, though symptom development may take some time. Suspect a chemical incident when you notice incapacitated small animals, birds, and insects. You may also be alerted to a possible chemical incident when confronted with chemical-exposure-like symptoms where chemicals are not usually used.

Identifying a biological agent at the time of release is probably impossible. There might be a cloud of dust or aerosolized material but there are no immediate signs and symptoms from those exposed. Such contamination also may be distributed by the mail or other mechanisms. The incident is likely to be recognized after the incubation period and only after several patients report to emergency departments or clinics with the disease. Then the local health department will investigate what all victims have in common to identify where the biological agent release took place. If you happen to notice many patients presenting with signs and symptoms of illness at or around the same time, consider a possible biological attack.

**4. Describe the characteristics of explosive, incendiary, nuclear, chemical, and biological weapons used in terrorism.**

### Explosive and incendiary agents

pp. 143–144

Explosives are the most likely method by which terrorists will strike. The bomb may range from a suicide bomber carrying a few sticks of dynamite to a large vehicle filled with highly explosive material. After the initial explosion, associated dangers include structural collapse, fire, electrical hazard, and combustible or toxic gas hazards. Also be wary of secondary explosives set intentionally to disrupt rescue and to injure emergency responders. After the blast, emergency responders are left to locate, extricate, and provide medical care for the victims.

Incendiary agents are a special subset of explosives with less explosive power and greater heat and burn potential. Some incendiary agents are of special concern. White phosphorus may spontaneously combust when exposed to air and may be a part of military munitions or a terrorist weapon. It can be very difficult to extinguish when it contacts the skin. Often, fire-resistant oil is used to exclude the air and extinguish any flame. Another example is magnesium, a metal that burns vigorously and at a high temperature (3,000°C). It also is difficult to extinguish. Incendiary agents are likely to cause severe and extensive burn injuries.

Terrorists may choose to increase the effectiveness of their weapons by incorporating other agents with explosives. In some cases, they surround the explosive charge with old auto batteries, thereby contaminating the explosion scene with both lead and sulfuric acid. They may also surround the charge with scrap metal, nails, or screws that act as shrapnel. In some cases in the Middle East, terrorists have surrounded the explosive with nails coated with a form of rat poison, a derivative of warfarin (Coumadin), to increase the severity of wound hemorrhage associated with shrapnel wounds.

### Nuclear

pp. 144–145

Nuclear detonation is the release of energy that is generated when heavy nuclei split (fission) or light nuclei combine (fusion) to form new elements. The unleashed energy is tremendous and creates an explosion of immense proportion. In addition to the extremes of the injury-producing mechanisms associated with conventional explosions, radiant heat is likely to incinerate everything in the immediate vicinity of the blast and induce serious burn injury to exposed skin even at great distances from the blast epicenter. Burn injuries are likely to be the most lethal and debilitating injuries associated with a nuclear detonation. The damage associated with a typical nuclear detonation is extreme and results in concentric circles of total destruction and mortality, severe destruction and very high mortality, heavy destruction and moderate mortality, and light destruction and limited mortality.

The explosive energy disrupts communications, power, water and waste service, travel, and the medical, emergency medical, and public safety infrastructures. The destruction also disrupts access to the scene and limits the ability of the EMS system to identify, reach, and care for the seriously injured. It is an extreme disaster with great loss of life and injury and presents a great challenge to emergency responders.

The nuclear reaction also generates particles of debris and dust that give off nuclear radiation. Gases, heated by the explosion, draw these particles high into the atmosphere, where upper air currents carry the contamination until it falls to earth as fallout. This uplifting of irradiated debris leaves the scene almost radiation free from moments after the blast until about 1 hour post-ignition. Thereafter, there is a serious danger from fallout at the scene and downwind for many, many miles.

Nuclear radiation cannot be felt, seen, or otherwise detected by any of our senses. However, it damages the cells of the human body as it passes through them. Radiation passage changes the structure of molecules and essential elements of the cells. Damaged cells then go on to repair themselves, to die, or to produce altered or damaged cells (cancer). As the intensity and duration of exposure increases, so do the degree and extent of cell damage and the risk to life. Nuclear radiation from the sun and other natural sources bombards us constantly. This exposure is very limited and the damage caused by it is minimal. However, the initial radiation produced by the nuclear chain reaction (the blast) and fallout can produce serious and life-threatening exposure.

©2013 Pearson Education, Inc.
*Paramedic Care: Principles & Practice, Vol. 7, 4th Ed.*

Radioactive contamination may also be spread using conventional explosives (the "dirty bomb"). This type of blast is of conventional origin and does not cause the great magnitude of destruction that a nuclear detonation would. However, the explosion distributes radioactive material over a large area and into the surrounding air. The result is an explosion site with radioactive material contaminating the immediate vicinity. The greatest danger of this terrorist weapon is that the nature of the risk (the radiation) may not be recognized until well after the incident. Consequently, many more individuals and rescuers may be exposed or contaminated.

## Chemical

pp. 145–148

Potential chemical weapons range from simple hazardous materials common in our society to sophisticated chemicals specifically designed to harm humans. Because these chemical weapons are often gases or aerosols that will disperse in an open or windy area, the more common targets for their use are confined spaces such as subways or large buildings, which have central heating or air conditioning, or areas where many people congregate, such as arenas, shopping malls, and convention centers.

Volatility is the ease with which a chemical changes from a liquid to a gas. A chemical that remains a liquid is said to be persistent and poses a contact or absorption threat, whereas vapors, gases, and aerosols present an inhalation danger. Specific gravity refers to the density or weight of the vapor or gas as compared with air. A vapor or gas with a specific gravity less than that of air rises and quickly disperses into the atmosphere. A gas with a specific gravity greater than that of air sinks beneath it, stays close to the ground, and accumulates in low places.

Chemical weapons are classified according to the way they cause damage to the human body. These chemicals include nerve agents, vesicants, pulmonary agents, biotoxins, incapacitating agents, and other hazardous chemicals.

**Nerve Agents.** Nerve agents and some insecticides damage nervous impulse conduction. These agents generally inhibit the degradation of a neurotransmitter (acetylcholine) and quickly cause a nervous system overload, resulting in muscle twitching and spasms, convulsions, unconsciousness, and respiratory failure.

Nerve agents present as either vapor or liquid and are capable of being absorbed through the skin or inhaled and absorbed through the respiratory system. Exposure quickly leads to a series of signs and symptoms that can be remembered as SLUDGE—salivation, lacrimation, urination, diarrhea, gastrointestinal distress, and emesis. In addition to these signs, the patient may experience dyspnea, fasciculations (these are prominent), rhinorrhea, blurry vision, miosis, nausea, and sweating. Ultimately, the patient may become unconscious, seize, stop breathing, and die.

**Vesicants (Blistering Agents).** Vesicants are agents that damage exposed tissue, frequently causing vesicles (blisters). They are capable of causing damage to the skin, eyes, respiratory tract, and lungs, and are able to induce generalized illness as well. With the exception of phosgene oxime, the vesicants are thick, oily liquids that create a toxic vapor threat in warm temperatures.

Patients exposed to vesicants present with the signs and symptoms of injury to the skin, mucous membranes, and lungs. Exposed skin exhibits the signs of a chemical burn, including pain, erythema, and eventually blistering. The eyes and upper airway display a burning or stinging sensation with tearing and rhinorrhea. Respiratory tract exposure results in dyspnea, cough, wheezing, and pulmonary edema. Systemic signs and symptoms include nausea, vomiting, and fatigue. Signs and symptoms occur slowly with the mustard agents, which may prolong exposure.

**Pulmonary Agents.** Pulmonary agents are those that cause chemical injury primarily to the lungs. These agents attack the mucous membranes of the respiratory system from the oral pharynx and nasal pharynx to the smaller respiratory bronchioles and alveoli. They produce inflammation and pulmonary edema, resulting in dyspnea and hypoxia. Early signs and symptoms of pulmonary agent exposure are related to irritation of the upper airway. They include rhinorrhea; nasal, oral, and throat irritation; wheezing; and cough. The victim may also experience tearing and eye irritation. Pulmonary edema is generally a late sign of exposure.

**Biotoxins.** Another type of agent that is classified as a biological agent but behaves more like a chemical agent is the biotoxin.

Ricin, a by-product of castor oil production, inhibits the body's ability to synthesize proteins. It may be either aerosolized and inhaled or ingested. Ricin causes pulmonary edema when inhaled and gastric symptoms when ingested. Poisoning by both routes may cause shock and multiple-organ failure.

Staphylococcal enterotoxin is produced by a bacterium, *Staphylococcus aureus*, and is the agent most commonly responsible for food poisoning. Contamination may occur either orally, causing nausea and vomiting, or by inhalation, causing dyspnea and fever.

Botulinum, the most toxic agent known, is an infrequent result of improper canning technique. Botulinum can be ingested or inhaled. Botulinum attacks the nervous system. It interferes with impulse transmission and interrupts the central nervous system's control of the organs. The result is weakness, paralysis, and death by respiratory failure.

Trichothecene mycotoxins are a group of biotoxins produced by fungus molds. They prohibit protein and nucleic acid formulation and affect body cells that divide rapidly first. T2 acts very quickly, causing skin irritation (pain, burning, redness, and blistering), respiratory irritation (nasal and oral pain, rhinorrhea, epistaxis, wheezing, dyspnea, and hemoptysis), eye irritation (pain, redness, tearing, and blurry vision), and gastrointestinal symptoms (nausea, vomiting, abdominal cramping, and bloody diarrhea). T2 is most effective when absorbed through the skin. Generalized signs and symptoms include central nervous system signs, hypotension, and death.

**Incapacitating Agents.** Incapacitating agents include the riot control agents used by police and for personal protection as well as newer agents being investigated by the military. These agents are intentionally selected or designed to incapacitate, not injure or harm, the recipient.

You may come into contact with these agents when they are released by police to suppress a large public disturbance or to subdue an assaultive or violent individual or are released by an individual for personal protection or possibly in the commission of a crime. These agents may, in the future, be used by those who wish to disrupt the public and incite terror.

The exposed patient often complains of eye irritation and tearing as well as rhinorrhea. If the agent is inhaled, these symptoms are often accompanied by airway irritation and dyspnea.

The anticholinergic agents (atropine-like drugs) BZ and QNB are the prototype incapacitating agents for the military. The primary method of distribution of these agents is through the detonation of a mixture of explosive and agent. This explosion produces an aerosolized cloud. Exposure to BZ and QNB produces inappropriate affect, dry mucous beds, dilated pupils, slurred speech, disorientation, blurred vision, inhibition of the sweating reflex, elevated body temperature, and facial flushing. These effects become apparent after about 30 minutes of inhalation and last for up to 8 hours. The most dangerous effects of exposure include dysrhythmias and hyperthermia from the loss of the sweating reflex. The actions of BZ and QNB may be reversed by the administration of physostigmine.

**Other Hazardous Chemicals.** Any toxic chemical has a potential for use as a weapon of mass destruction. Industry produces countless hazardous materials with the potential to cause great harm if released into the air or water supply or ignited to release toxic gases. The only difference between an accidental release and one that is intended to incite terror is that the intentional release will likely be optimized to affect the greatest number of people.

## Biological
pp. 148–150

Biological agents are either living organisms or toxins produced by living organisms that are deliberately distributed to cause disease, incapacitation, and death. Generally, these agents are grouped as noncontagious (anthrax and biotoxins) or as contagious and capable of spreading from human to human (smallpox, Ebola, plague). Contagious agents are of greatest concern because the people originally infected can spread the disease, often before the medical community has recognized that a biological weapon attack has occurred. EMS and other medical systems are especially vulnerable because they are called to treat those who first display the disease's signs and symptoms, possibly before the nature and significance of the disease is known. Noncontagious agents affect only those who received the initial dose, thus limiting the scope of the disease and making it somewhat easier to identify when and where the contact took place.

Mutant strains of common diseases such as the more serious variations of influenza, multiple-drug-resistant strains of tuberculosis, or the recent cold-like virus called severe acute respiratory syndrome (SARS) may emerge and create epidemics of massive proportions. Outbreaks of naturally occurring disease may be more likely and more severe than a terrorist's use of a biological weapon. Tracking the

©2013 Pearson Education, Inc.
*Paramedic Care: Principles & Practice, Vol. 7, 4th Ed.*

origin and combating these naturally occurring diseases is exactly like tracking and combating a biological weapon used by terrorists.

Currently the list of potential weapons of mass destruction (WMD) diseases is extensive and contains pneumonia-like agents, encephalitis-like agents, and others.

**Pneumonia-like Agents.** Pneumonia-like bioterror agents include anthrax, plague, tularemia, and Q fever and are the most likely agents for a terrorist attack. They generally cause cough, dyspnea, fever, and malaise. Anthrax and plague are the most deadly, with 90 to 100 percent mortality.

Anthrax is a very effective biological agent, though it is not contagious, which limits any human-to-human transmission.

The strain of plague most likely used for bioterrorism is pneumonic, which carries not only a very high mortality (100 percent untreated and about 57 percent when treated), but also has minimum victim survival when left untreated for the first 18 hours after signs and symptoms appear. Pneumonic plague incubates over 1 to 4 days and can be spread through droplets and inhalation.

Tularemia (also known as rabbit fever or deerfly fever) may be aerosolized and presents with signs and symptoms in 2 to 10 days. It carries a mortality rate of up to 5 percent.

Q fever may appear in 10 to 20 days after contact and lasts from 2 days to 2 weeks; however, it is more of an incapacitating disease with a very low death rate.

**Encephalitis-like Agents.** Smallpox and Venezuelan equine encephalitis (VEE) are influenza-like diseases with headache, fever, and malaise and a higher mortality, probably because these diseases attack the central nervous system. They are very effective as biological weapons because small amounts of aerosolized agent can cause the disease.

Smallpox is very contagious through airborne droplets via the respiratory route. Signs and symptoms usually appear after about 12 days in about 30 percent of those exposed, with about a third of that number dying within 5 to 7 days. Smallpox is considered eradicated as a naturally occurring disease, but it is thought that it may exist in the WMD programs of some countries.

With VEE, human-to-human transmission does not occur, and mortality is generally less than 20 percent.

**Other Agents.** Cholera is a common disease in underdeveloped countries and is frequently linked to poor sanitation. It is most commonly transmitted by the fecal–oral route and primarily causes severe dehydration and shock because of profuse diarrhea. It is one of the few agents that is not transmitted by the inhalation route and may be delivered as a weapon by way of contamination of food or untreated water.

Viral hemorrhagic fever (VHF) is a class of diseases that includes the deadly Ebola virus. As the name suggests, hemorrhagic fever attacks the bloodstream and damages blood vessels, causing them to leak and the patient to bleed easily. The patient may bruise easily and display petechiae. Most diseases of this class can be spread through the inhalation route or through direct contact with infectious material. VHFs may carry a high mortality rate (90 percent) and are aerosolized easily, though they are difficult to cultivate.

5. **Be aware of the likelihood of secondary explosions when responding to reports of an explosion.**                                                              pp. 143–144

Be wary of secondary explosives set intentionally to disrupt rescue and to injure emergency responders. Terrorists often set secondary explosive devices with the intent to disrupt any rescue attempt. They may set secondary detonations through booby traps or timers that are designed to target rescuers.

6. **Predict injury patterns and patient problems associated with explosions and the use of incendiary devices.**                                                 p. 143

The blast pressure wave causes compression/decompression injury as it passes through the lungs, the ears, and other hollow, air-filled organs. This damage may be enhanced when the explosion occurs in a confined space, such as the interior of a building or other structure. Debris thrown by the blast produces penetrating or blunt injuries, and similar additional injury occurs as the victim is thrown by the blast wind. Secondary combustion induces burn injury, and structural collapse causes blunt and crushing injuries.

**7. Describe the precautions in responding to a nuclear incident.** p. 145

The first hour post-ignition is generally spent moving the injured into structures that will protect them from fallout. Ideally, they are moved into the central areas of large, structurally sound buildings or at least to some cover from the falling contaminated dust. During this time, evacuation of those in the anticipated path of fallout occurs. They should remain outside the fallout pathway for at least 48 hours and until radiologic monitoring determines it is safe to return. Entry into the scene is made from upwind and laterally to upper air movement in order to limit radioactive fallout exposure to rescuers.

As the response is organized, egress and evacuation routes are cleared, the injured are located and evacuated, and the response moves closer and closer to the blast epicenter. In general, some limited medical care is provided where the victims are found, but most emergency medical care is provided at treatment sectors that are remote from the seriously damaged areas and away from where fallout is expected. Patients are brought to a decontamination area, monitored for contamination, and decontaminated as needed before care begins. A properly decontaminated patient does not pose a radiation threat either to himself or to you.

During a response to a suspected nuclear incident, you will likely wear a dosimeter, a pen-like device used to record your total radiation exposure. This device is then monitored to determine when your exposure level is such that you should leave the scene for your own safety. Specially trained scene responders or health physicists will monitor dosages and determine how long you, as a care provider, can safely work at the scene.

If the risk of fallout and continuing radiation exposure is serious, paramedics may be asked to help distribute potassium iodide (KI) tablets. These tablets reduce the uptake of radioactive iodine (a common component of radioactive fallout) by the thyroid, which reduces the risk of thyroid injury or cancer. You may also be involved in the effort to evacuate the public from the expected fallout path.

**8. Anticipate the patient presentations and risks to responders associated with chemical agent exposures.** p. 148

A chemical weapon release may be visible as a cloud of mist, vapor, dust, or as puddles, or it may be completely unrecognizable. There may be an associated smell such as that of newly mown grass (phosgene), the smell of rotten eggs (hydrogen sulfide), or other strange or unusual odors. Suspect a chemical release if there are chemical odors when and where chemicals are not used or expected. However, never search out such an odor or touch any suspect liquid or material. You may also notice clusters of patients with chemical exposure symptoms or injured, incapacitated, or dead insects, birds, or animals. Given that the terrorist may be intent on optimizing the effect of the release, be especially wary of large public gatherings or large but confined spaces such as a public buildings and low spaces that limit dissipation such as subway terminals. Terrorists may also target food or water supplies with either chemical or biological agents. This may result in very widespread effects.

A cardinal sign of a chemical release is the manifestation of similar signs and symptoms occurring rapidly among a group of individuals. Common signs of a chemical release include inflamed mucosa (eye, nasal, oral, or throat irritation), exposed skin irritation, chest tightness, burning and/or dyspnea, gastrointestinal signs (nausea, abdominal cramping, vomiting, and diarrhea) and central nervous system disturbances (confusion, lethargy, nausea/vomiting, intoxication, headache, and unconsciousness).

Approach the scene from upwind and higher ground and remain a good distance away from the site. Generally, evacuate the immediate area if the release is small and contained. However, if the release involves a great quantity of material, such as that in a railway tank car or large commercial storage container, evacuate the general population for a radius of 700 to 2,000 feet and 1.5 miles downwind during the day. If the release occurs at night, then evacuate a 2,000-foot radius and as much as 6 to 7 miles downwind.

Once the public danger is reduced by scene isolation, make sure the injured are properly decontaminated before you begin care. Rescuers coming out of the danger zones must also be decontaminated. The agency that provides spill containment and decontamination at the hazardous materials incident generally provides decontamination for both nuclear and chemical weapons of mass destruction.

In addition to the specific emergency care steps, most patients require decontamination, exposure to fresh air, oxygen administration, and possibly respiratory support. As a precautionary measure, use personal protective equipment (PPE), including a well-fitting HEPA filter mask, nitrile gloves (latex

©2013 Pearson Education, Inc.
*Paramedic Care: Principles & Practice, Vol. 7, 4th Ed.*

gloves do not offer much protection against chemical agents), and a Tyvek® disposable suit. Be careful of leather clothing items. Belts, watch bands, and shoes made of leather absorb many chemical agents and will present a continuing exposure danger once contaminated. These precautions provide very minimal protection against chemical agents and do not constitute the PPE necessary to work in a warm or hot zone.

9. **Describe the specific treatment for chemical agent exposures.**

### Nerve agents
p. 146

The actions of nerve agents can generally be reversed if the antidote is administered shortly after exposure. However, many nerve agents permanently bind to the agents, reabsorbing the neurotransmitters, and their effects become more difficult to reverse. The prognosis for a patient exposed to a nerve agent is good with aggressive artificial ventilation and quick administration of the antidote.

Treatment for nerve agent exposure includes the administration of atropine and then pralidoxime chloride. The military currently has these medications available in a two-part auto-injector set called a Mark I kit. The auto-injectors are designed for self-administration or buddy administration (mainly for military personnel) or may be administered by rescue personnel. They are quick to use and may be necessary when confronted with numerous patients exposed to a nerve agent. The antidote combination is often followed by the administration of diazepam to reduce seizure activity. The auto-injector is a convenient way to administer this regimen of medications; however, the intravenous route is more rapid and preferred when available and as time permits.

The Mark I kit contains 2 mg of atropine and 600 mg of pralidoxime chloride. It is administered for the first and mild symptoms of exposure (blurry vision, mild dyspnea, and rhinorrhea) and repeated in 10 minutes if symptoms do not improve. If serious signs and symptoms are present, three doses of both atropine and pralidoxime chloride may be administered. Intravenous administration should provide 2 mg of atropine every 5 minutes (until drying of secretions or 20 mg is administered) and 1 g of pralidoxime chloride every hour (until spontaneous respirations return). A pediatric version of the Mark I kit is available.

### Vesicants (blistering agents)
pp. 146–147

Emergency care for the patient exposed to a vesicant is immediate decontamination. Exposure of even a few minutes can result in permanent injury. The exposed areas should be irrigated immediately with water from a hose (using limited pressure if possible). Also irrigate the eyes, with a preference for saline over water, but do not delay irrigation to await the proper fluid. If blistering has occurred, treat the lesions as you would any chemical burn. Apply loose sterile dressings, gently bandage affected eyes, and medicate the patient for any serious pain.

### Pulmonary agents
p. 147

Emergency care for the individual exposed to a pulmonary agent is removal from the environment; exposure to fresh air; high-flow, high-concentration oxygen; and rest. Endotracheal intubation and ventilation may be required. In cases of moderate to severe respiratory distress, consider 0.5 mL of albuterol by nebulized inhalation.

### Biotoxins
p. 147

Management of a victim of a biotoxin is supportive; antitoxins are generally not available. A special concern is directed to careful decontamination because even a very small amount of biotoxin can endanger rescuers and others.

### Incapacitating agents
pp. 147–148

Signs and symptoms are relieved by removal from the source, exposure to fresh air, and the administration of oxygen, when needed. The signs and symptoms further diminish with time.

### Other hazardous chemicals
p. 148

It may also be more difficult to identify the agent used by a terrorist because the container will likely not identify the agent. The Department of Transportation's *Emergency Response Guidebook*, which should be carried on every ambulance and fire apparatus, is a good guide to most common hazardous materials that might be used as a weapon as well as information on other WMD agents. It can also be helpful in denoting isolation and evacuation distances and suggesting specific care management steps.

**10. Describe the keys to recognizing a biological terrorist attack.** pp. 148–149

Identification of a biological agent release is difficult because there is often no noticeable cloud of gas or any noticeable odor. This identification is especially challenging because any signs and symptoms of the disease occur at the end of the incubation period, often days or weeks after the initial contact. Rapid identification is further complicated because many potential biological weapons present with signs and symptoms typical of influenza or many other common and general illnesses.

Most commonly, the existence of a biological attack is recognized when numerous patients report to the emergency department or medical clinic with similar signs and symptoms or when a health care provider notices a geographic cluster of patients. Care providers may also notice a disease occurring out of season (many patients with flu-like symptoms during the summer) or a disease outside its normal geographic regions (tropical disease in the northern latitudes). Only then can the health department begin to work to identify the disease's nature and when and where the exposure most likely happened. By the time the disease outbreak is recognized as a bioterrorism event, secondary exposures from those affected by contagious agents may already be occurring. These secondary exposures may include family members, friends, workmates, and the medical system, including EMS, emergency department personnel, and other health care providers.

**11. Describe the specific actions to be taken by responders to protect themselves when responding to a biological terrorist attack.** pp. 150–151

Protection against the most common biological weapons includes the prudent care steps used to prevent ordinary communicable disease transmission. If there is a heightened alert status for a WMD release or terrorist event, employ a more aggressive use of Standard Precautions. Gloves are very effective in protecting against biological agent transmission from body fluids, as is rigorous and frequent hand washing. Almost all biological agents are transmitted by the respiratory route, so be sure to take droplet inhalation precautions. A properly fitted HEPA respirator is very effective in preventing agent transmission. Consider applying a mask to your patient if he displays any signs or symptoms of respiratory disease. A sodium hypochlorite solution (0.5 percent) or other disinfectants are very effective in killing many biological agents. The ambulance interior and any equipment used or possibly contaminated should be vigorously cleaned with the solution.

Immunizations against many biological agents are not available. Those immunizations that are available usually carry a small risk of associated reaction. Hence, the prophylactic administration to a very large number of health care workers may not be warranted unless or until a significant risk becomes apparent.

The public health approach to biological terrorism may also involve isolation and quarantine. The patient or caregiver exposed to a highly contagious disease may be quarantined through a restriction to home or may be confined within a commandeered facility such as a motel. A person with the signs and symptoms of the disease may be isolated through a similar arrangement. There is a danger associated with placing affected patients or caregivers in a hospital or other medical facility because they can then endanger other patients or care providers who are receiving or providing care there.

# Case Study Review

*Reread the case study on page 142 in* Paramedic Care: Operations; *then, read the following discussion.*
*This case study illustrates how the events of September 11, 2001, have affected EMS professionals and their responsibilities. It highlights the need to include the possibility of terrorist acts in all aspects of emergency care decision making.*

Adam and Sean have a heightened index of suspicion for a weapon of mass destruction incident that comes following the events of September 11, 2001. When presented with several patients with similar symptoms, they suspect a chemical agent release and request activation of the country's WMD plan. They also approach the scene with care, arriving upwind of the building and directing dispatch to request evacuation (thereby evacuating the building without risk to rescuers). Sean and Adam also request the fire department (their local hazmat team) to respond as well. Finally, by using a cell phone rather than using the EMS radio, they assure their suspicion of a WMD incident is not made public.

Adam and Sean direct the potential patients to their care station using the public address system, again reducing any risk to the rescuers. They establish incident management and effectively communicate pertinent information regarding the numbers and types of patients they are encountering. This helps the emergency department prepare for the arrival of numerous patients with the same complaints. Before stepping from their rig, Sean and Adam don HEPA-filter masks and gloves to further protect themselves from any biological threat.

Adam relinquishes incident management responsibilities as soon as someone from the fire department arrives. He communicates his knowledge of the scene and then joins Sean in treating the patients. Because the number of patients outnumbers the resources available, Sean and Adam provide oxygen only to the most seriously affected patients. Thankfully, the symptoms are only minor and other ambulances arrive quickly. As more information is gathered about the scene, the initial information suggests a simple furnace or chimney malfunction. However, further investigation suggests that this was truly a WMD incident involving the intentional production of carbon monoxide. The scene then becomes a crime scene and is investigated thoroughly by the police department.

# Content Self-Evaluation

## MULTIPLE CHOICE

_____ 1. Which of the following is the most likely weapon of choice for terrorist groups?
   A. Conventional explosives
   B. Nuclear weapons
   C. Biological agents
   D. Chemical agents
   E. Incendiary devices

_____ 2. Terrorists are likely to target which of the following?
   A. An embassy
   B. A symbol of government
   C. Their employer
   D. Corporations
   E. All of the above

_____ 3. The blast pressure wave is likely to injure all of the following, EXCEPT the
   A. lungs.
   B. ears.
   C. bowel.
   D. heart.
   E. sinuses.

_____ 4. After the initial explosion, associated dangers include all of the following, EXCEPT
   A. electrical hazards
   B. inability to recognize the incident.
   C. fire.
   D. structural collapse.
   E. toxic hazards.

_____ 5. Incendiary agents differ from conventional explosives in that they
   A. have greater explosive energy.
   B. cause more burn injuries.
   C. consume more oxygen.
   D. are dropped from a high altitude.
   E. combine both explosive and nuclear damage.

_____ 6. The best way to detect radiation in the absence of a Geiger counter is by
   A. a strange taste in your mouth.
   B. a warm sensation in your muscles.
   C. immediate nausea.
   D. a tingling sensation from the exposed surface.
   E. none of the above.

7. Which of the following is the mechanism of injury associated with most deaths from a nuclear blast?
   A. Radiation burns
   B. Radiation illness
   C. Cancer
   D. Thermal burns
   E. Pressure injuries

8. Fallout associated with nuclear detonation is not likely to be a factor until how long after the detonation?
   A. 10 minutes
   B. 30 minutes
   C. 1 hour
   D. 4 hours
   E. 2 days

9. Once a victim exposed to nuclear radiation and debris has been properly decontaminated, he poses no danger to himself or others.
   A. True
   B. False

10. Which of the following is a symptom associated with radiation exposure?
    A. Nausea
    B. Fatigue
    C. Malaise
    D. Hypertension
    E. All of the above except D

11. Which of the following influence(s) the delivery of a chemical weapon?
    A. Wind strength
    B. The agent's specific gravity
    C. The agent's volatility
    D. Precipitation
    E. All of the above

12. Which of the following is NOT a common sign or symptom of a nerve agent?
    A. Dry mouth
    B. Tearing eyes
    C. Urination
    D. Defecation
    E. Vomiting

13. Blistering agents are also known as
    A. organophosphates.
    B. vesicants.
    C. carbamates.
    D. chambering agents.
    E. none of the above.

14. Which of the following is NOT a blistering agent?
    A. Lewisite
    B. Phosgene oxime
    C. Botulinum
    D. Sulfur mustard
    E. Nitrogen mustard

15. One of the most toxic agents known to man is
    A. sulfur mustard.
    B. ricin.
    C. VX gas.
    D. botulinum.
    E. none of the above.

16. Which of the following suggests a chemical agent release?
    A. A strange smell
    B. Numerous patients complaining of the same symptoms
    C. A cloud of dust or gas
    D. Incapacitated or dead birds and insects
    E. All of the above

17. Which of the following is NOT a biological agent capable of spreading from person-to-person?
    A. Ebola
    B. Smallpox
    C. Plague
    D. Anthrax
    E. Cholera

©2013 Pearson Education, Inc.
*Paramedic Care: Principles & Practice, Vol. 7, 4th Ed.*

_____ 18. A biological release can be recognized by which of the following?
   A.  A distinctive cloud
   B.  A distinctive color
   C.  Immediate signs and symptoms
   D.  Very distinct signs and symptoms
   E.  None of the above

_____ 19. The most likely biological agents to be used by terrorists are
   A.  pneumonia-like agents.
   B.  flu-like agents.
   C.  encephalitis-like agents.
   D.  Ebola.
   E.  all of the above.

_____ 20. Almost all biological weapons are transmitted via the respiratory route; therefore, the HEPA respirator is very effective at reducing transmission.
   A.  True
   B.  False

# Special Project

## Nerve Agent Awareness

**Part I**

_The signs and symptoms of nerve agent exposure can be remembered by using the mnemonic "SLUGDE." On the lines below, identify each of the SLUDGE components._

S  _____

L  _____

U  _____

D  _____

G  _____

E  _____

**Part II**

_A Mark I kit is a two-part auto-injector set used to treat nerve agent exposure. What two medications are included in the kit?_

_____

_____

# OPERATIONS
# Content Review
## *Content Self-Evaluation*

## Chapter 1: Ground Ambulance Operations

_____ 1. Reasons for routine inspection of the ambulance and equipment include all of the following, EXCEPT
  A. ensuring that equipment is ready and available.
  B. ensuring that the work environment is safe.
  C. reminding personnel where all supplies are.
  D. ensuring the cleanliness of the ambulance.
  E. evaluating the performance of other paramedics.

_____ 2. Responsibility for reporting ambulance or equipment problems lies with
  A. inspectors for the local, regional, or state EMS offices.
  B. the paramedic who identifies the problem.
  C. the paramedic or responder on the next shift.
  D. the supervisor responsible for vehicles or supplies.
  E. none of the above.

_____ 3. Maneuvering ambulances and crews in an effort to reduce response times is a strategy known as
  A. deployment.                      D. peak load response.
  B. reserve capacity.                E. tiered response.
  C. system status management.

_____ 4. The term for the ability of an EMS agency to respond to calls beyond those handled by the on-duty crews is called
  A. deployment.                      D. peak load response.
  B. reserve capacity.                E. tiered response.
  C. system status management.

_____ 5. Based on the statistics from New York, the profile of a typical ambulance collision is
  A. a lateral collision that takes place on a dry road during daylight hours on a clear day in an intersection without a traffic light.
  B. a lateral collision that takes place on a wet road during daylight hours on a rainy day in an intersection with a traffic light.
  C. a lateral collision that takes place on a wet road during daylight hours on a clear day in an intersection with a traffic light.
  D. a lateral collision that takes place on a dry road during daylight hours on a clear day in an intersection with a traffic light.
  E. a lateral collision that takes place on a wet road during nighttime hours on a clear day in an intersection without a traffic light.

_____ 6. According to recent studies, motorists do not hear sirens or see emergency lights until the ambulance is within
  A. 50 feet or less.                 D. 50 to 100 yards.
  B. 50 to 100 feet.                  E. 100 to 150 yards.
  C. 100 to 150 feet.

_____ 7. If there are no fire or escaping liquids or fumes, park the ambulance at least
   A. 25 feet from the wreckage.          D. 100 feet from the wreckage.
   B. 50 feet from the wreckage.          E. 125 feet from the wreckage.
   C. 75 feet from the wreckage.

_____ 8. Remember that lights and siren only "ask" the public to yield the right of way.
   A. True.
   B. False.

# Chapter 2: Air Medical Operations

_____ 9. In Korea, patients were evacuated from the battlefield to a
   A. Medical Army Surgical Hospital.
   B. Mobile Army Specialty Hospital.
   C. Medical Army Specialty Hospital.
   D. Mobile Army Surgical Hospital.
   E. Mobile Armored Surgical Hospital.

_____ 10. One of the most significant limitations that all helicopters face is the
   A. size of landing zone.
   B. weather.
   C. time of day.
   D. weight of crew and patient.
   E. none of the above.

_____ 11. The choice of aircraft type is usually based on all the following, EXCEPT
   A. patient condition.
   B. medical needs.
   C. distance of transport.
   D. patient preference.
   E. availability.

_____ 12. Which of the following is NOT an appropriate reason to use an air medical helicopter in the out-of-hospital setting?
   A. The patient has a significant potential to require a time-critical intervention and an air medical helicopter will deliver the patient to an appropriate facility faster than ground transport.
   B. Local EMS resources are exceeded.
   C. The patient has a significant potential to require high-level life support available from an air medical helicopter, which is not available by ground transport.
   D. The patient's insurance provides coverage for air medical services.
   E. The patient is located in a geographically isolated area that would make ground transport impossible or greatly delayed.

_____ 13. All of the following are crew configurations EXCEPT
   A. paramedic and nurse.
   B. basic and paramedic.
   C. paramedic and specialist.
   D. nurse and physician.
   E. paramedic and paramedic.

©2013 Pearson Education, Inc.
*Paramedic Care: Principles & Practice, Vol. 7, 4th Ed.*

14. The Paramedic First Air Ambulance Alliance (PFAA) is a grassroots organization committed to ensuring that critically ill and injured patients have access to the safest and highest-quality air medical system possible.
   A. True
   B. False

15. The easiest strobes to be seen at night if the pilot is using night vision goggles are
   A. red and white.
   B. green and white.
   C. blue and green.
   D. blue and white.
   E. red and blue.

16. All of the following are components of "HOTSAW," EXCEPT
   A. animals.
   B. terrain.
   C. hazards.
   D. space.
   E. wind.

17. The flight crew will typically want you to bring them the patient as soon they indicate it is safe.
   A. True.
   B. False.

18. If an ambulance is used to move the patient to the aircraft, it should never get closer than
   A. 10 feet to the aircraft.
   B. 15 feet to the aircraft.
   C. 20 feet to the aircraft.
   D. 25 feet to the aircraft.
   E. 30 feet to the aircraft.

# Chapter 3: Multiple-Casualty Incidents and Incident Management

19. The IMS currently used by the emergency response system originated from
   A. the Southern California fire service.
   B. the federal Department of Transportation.
   C. OSHA.
   D. the National Incident Management System.
   E. the Homeland Security Administration.

20. What event served as the precipitating impetus for development of a national incident management program?
   A. California wildfires
   B. Terrorist attacks in 2001
   C. Anthrax letters
   D. Reorganization of the National Fire Service
   E. All of the above

21. The C-FLOP mnemonic identifies the five elements of the incident management system. The "P" stands for which of the following?
   A. Patient assessment
   B. Political coordination
   C. Planning
   D. Preemptive action
   E. Past experience

_____ 22. Generally, the IMS would be implemented in which of these situations?
- A. When an ambulance is deployed to an MVC
- B. At the scene of a technical rescue operation
- C. At the scene of a traumatic cardiac arrest
- D. When two or more units respond to an incident
- E. All of the above

_____ 23. Managers from different jurisdictions for law enforcement, fire, and EMS coordinate their activities and share responsibility for command through a process known as
- A. unified command.
- B. ultimate authority.
- C. singular command.
- D. span of control.
- E. none of the above.

_____ 24. The officers who perform supervisory roles in the IMS rather than those who actually perform a task are called
- A. section chiefs.
- B. management staff.
- C. staff function officers.
- D. demobilizing officers.
- E. medical officers.

_____ 25. Monitoring the emotional status of all on-scene personnel and providing support as needed is the job of the
- A. management staff.
- B. agency chaplain.
- C. command staff.
- D. mental health support.
- E. incident commander.

_____ 26. Which of the following units is NOT usually under EMS branch authority at a typical multiple-casualty incident?
- A. Triage
- B. Treatment
- C. Transport
- D. Decontamination
- E. Staging

_____ 27. At the disaster, which patients are collected at the morgue?
- A. Emergent
- B. Delayed
- C. Expectant
- D. Minimal
- E. Both B and C

_____ 28. The IMS unit responsible for monitoring and supporting on-scene responders is the
- A. extrication unit.
- B. scene safety officer.
- C. triage sector.
- D. rehabilitation unit.
- E. staging unit.

# Chapter 4: Rescue Awareness and Operations

_____ 29. Which of the following is NOT considered a special rescue operation?
- A. Low-head dam
- B. High-angle rescue
- C. Confined-space rescue
- D. Cardiac arrest
- E. Vehicle rescue

_____ 30. Every rescue operation should have a safety officer who has the knowledge and authority to intervene in unsafe situations.
- A. True
- B. False

©2013 Pearson Education, Inc.
_Paramedic Care: Principles & Practice, Vol. 7, 4th Ed._

_____ **31.** General phases of rescue operations include
   **A.** disentanglement.
   **B.** packaging.
   **C.** hazard control.
   **D.** size-up.
   **E.** all of the above.

_____ **32.** When approaching a rescue scene, your scene size-up should provide you with information about
   **A.** the nature of the situation.
   **B.** scene safety and hazards.
   **C.** the total number of victims.
   **D.** the need for special rescue teams.
   **E.** all of the above.

_____ **33.** Initial responding units often overestimate their capability to handle a rescue situation or are hesitant to request reserves or specialty teams.
   **A.** True
   **B.** False

_____ **34.** Care for an entrapped patient during a lengthy rescue differs from normal patient care because it involves
   **A.** greater patient stabilization skills.
   **B.** more psychological support for the patient.
   **C.** protection from a more hostile environment.
   **D.** protection from extended rescue operations.
   **E.** all of the above.

_____ **35.** Water immersion causes body heat to be lost how many times faster than air?
   **A.** 2
   **B.** 10
   **C.** 15
   **D.** 25
   **E.** 40

_____ **36.** Factors that contribute to drowning associated with cool or cold water immersion include which of the following?
   **A.** Inability to self-rescue
   **B.** Laryngospasm
   **C.** Inability to grasp a line
   **D.** Inability to follow simple directions
   **E.** All of the above

_____ **37.** The proper order for the water rescue method is which of the following?
   **A.** Row-throw-go-reach
   **B.** Reach-throw-row-go
   **C.** Throw-go-reach-row
   **D.** Go-throw-reach-row
   **E.** Row-throw-reach-go

_____ **38.** The longest cold water submersion that resulted in successful resuscitation was for what length of time?
   **A.** 10 minutes
   **B.** 45 minutes
   **C.** Just over an hour
   **D.** 2 ½ hours
   **E.** 4 hours

_____ **39.** Who is the most likely victim of a hazardous atmosphere?
   **A.** A farmer
   **B.** An industrial worker
   **C.** An excavator
   **D.** A petroleum or chemical plant worker
   **E.** A rescuer

_____ **40.** The greatest hazard associated with motor vehicle collisions is which of the following?
   **A.** Traffic flow
   **B.** Spilled fuel
   **C.** Spilled toxic chemicals (battery acid)
   **D.** Glass
   **E.** Jagged metal

_____ **41.** The electrical systems of hybrid electric vehicles contain a
      **A.** low-voltage and a 12-volt battery.
      **B.** high-voltage and a 12-volt battery.
      **C.** high-voltage and a 24-volt battery.
      **D.** low-voltage and a 12-volt battery.
      **E.** high-voltage and a 6-volt battery.

_____ **42.** The term that describes descending by sliding down a fixed double rope is
      **A.** belaying.                 **D.** controlled descent.
      **B.** dynamic anchoring.      **E.** high-angle scrambling.
      **C.** rappelling.

_____ **43.** Extended care issues that need specific protocols include which of the following?
      **A.** Long-term hydration management      **D.** Hyperthemia management
      **B.** Removal of impaled objects          **E.** All of the above
      **C.** Wound cleansing

# Chapter 5: Hazardous Materials Incidents

_____ **44.** Priorities for a hazmat incident are the same as for any other major incident: life safety, incident stabilization, and property conservation.
      **A.** True
      **B.** False

_____ **45.** Paramedics should suspect hazardous material involvement at a(n)
      **A.** overturned tractor-trailer.      **D.** explosion at a government office.
      **B.** fire alarm at a hospital.         **E.** all of the above.
      **C.** collision at a railroad crossing.

_____ **46.** Chemical, biological, or nuclear devices used by terrorists to strike at government or high-profile targets are called
      **A.** clandestine weapons of terror.
      **B.** international weapons of ruin.
      **C.** weapons of mass destruction.
      **D.** domestic implements of war.
      **E.** weapons of motivational destruction.

_____ **47.** A four-digit identification number specific to a given chemical is a(n)
      **A.** NFPA code.              **D.** IDLH.
      **B.** UN number.            **E.** bill of lading.
      **C.** U.S. number.

_____ **48.** An example of a computer-aided database used for hazmat references and operations is the
      **A.** CAMEO.              **D.** Canadian material sort system.
      **B.** UN computer system.     **E.** _Emergency Response Guidebook._
      **C.** MSDS database.

_____ **49.** Which of the following zones is associated with and contains the primary contamination at the hazardous materials incident?
      **A.** Red zone              **D.** Blue zone
      **B.** Yellow zone         **E.** Black zone
      **C.** Green zone

©2013 Pearson Education, Inc.
_Paramedic Care: Principles & Practice, Vol. 7, 4th Ed._

_____ 50. The lowest temperature at which a chemical will give off enough vapor to ignite is the
A. boiling point.
B. flash point.
C. flammable limit.
D. ignition temperature.
E. vapor pressure.

_____ 51. The radiation capable of traveling only a few inches through air is
A. alpha.
B. beta.
C. gamma.
D. neutron.
E. X-ray.

_____ 52. The only poisoning where the administration of ipecac is appropriate to induce vomiting is for severe corrosive ingestion.
A. True
B. False

_____ 53. The level of hazmat protection worn by firefighters and not suitable for hazmat situations is
A. level A.
B. level B.
C. level C.
D. level D.
E. level E.

# Chapter 6: Crime Scene Awareness

_____ 54. The age group with the highest arrest rates for violent crimes is which of the following?
A. 0 to 10 years of age
B. 10 to 14 years of age
C. 15 to 34 years of age
D. 35 to 50 years of age
E. 50 years and older

_____ 55. Bullying is a form of youth violence and can result in
A. emotional distress.
B. death.
C. social distress.
D. physical injury.
E. all of the above.

_____ 56. In most cases, you can legally leave a patient behind when there is a documented danger.
A. True
B. False

_____ 57. A crime that is committed against a person solely on the basis of the individual's religion is an example of
A. assault and battery.
B. a federal crime.
C. a crime of passion.
D. a hate crime.
E. a racist act.

_____ 58. One of the most common substances manufactured in drug laboratories is
A. marijuana.
B. methamphetamine.
C. date-rape drugs.
D. opiate narcotics.
E. methadone.

_____ 59. All of the following are safety tactics the paramedic could use in a dangerous situation, EXCEPT
A. retreat.
B. cover and concealment.
C. distraction and evasion.
D. camouflage and cover.
E. contact and cover.

_____ 60. EMS personnel trained to serve with a tactical EMS or a law enforcement agency are called:
A. EMT-Swats.
B. SWATEMs.
C. EMT-TEMs.
D. EMT-Tacticals.
E. CONTOMs.

_____ 61. Clothing samples should be placed in a clear plastic bag when taken from the crime scene, as this prevents contamination from chemicals in the air.
  A. True
  B. False

_____ 62. Exam gloves prevent you from leaving print evidence at the scene and reduce the chances of you smudging prints left by others.
  A. True
  B. False

_____ 63. Blood splatter evidence is important because it helps identify
  A. the type of weapon used.
  B. the position of the attacker in relation to the victim.
  C. the direction of the attack.
  D. the force of the attack.
  E. all of the above.

# Chapter 7: Rural EMS

_____ 64. Rural residents suffer a higher level of mortality associated with medical emergencies because
  A. there are greater distances to health care.
  B. of a lack of experienced EMS providers.
  C. helicopter transport is overutilized.
  D. rural residents are sicker to begin with.
  E. of a lack of adequately equipped ambulances.

_____ 65. A term for an inability to keep abreast of new technologies and standards is
  A. lost opportunity.          D. poor management.
  B. block out.                 E. deficient networking.
  C. rust out.

_____ 66. Communication difficulties are a major problem in rural areas simply because of a lack of cell phone coverage.
  A. True
  B. False

_____ 67. Facilities that provide limited care and nonemergent medical treatment are
  A. fast tracks.               D. prompt care facilities.
  B. "docs in a box."           E. health care outreaches.
  C. rural hostels.

_____ 68. Which of the following would you expect to be thinly distributed in the rural or wilderness setting?
  A. Full-service hospitals     D. Physicians
  B. Fire service               E. All of the above
  C. EMS units

_____ 69. Rural emergency care is likely to cause which of the following changes to the normal EMS response?
  A. less dependable detection
  B. longer response times to the scene
  C. longer transport times
  D. less dependable physician availability at rural hospitals
  E. all of the above

©2013 Pearson Education, Inc.
_Paramedic Care: Principles & Practice, Vol. 7, 4th Ed._

_____ **70.** Hazards associated with agricultural activities include which of the following?
  **A.** Machinery entrapment
  **B.** Hazardous materials
  **C.** Entombment under grain or silage
  **D.** Confined space/toxic environment
  **E.** All of the above

_____ **71.** The procedure that calls for turning equipment off and marking it so it is not turned on is called
  **A.** positive lock out.          **D.** lock-out/tag-out.
  **B.** definitive shutdown.         **E.** none of the above.
  **C.** keyed/disabled.

_____ **72.** Which of the following is an advantage to using an EMS helicopter in a rural or wilderness area?
  **A.** Transport is less expensive.
  **B.** They are available in all types of weather.
  **C.** It is rare that a helicopter will not be available.
  **D.** They can travel quickly over rough terrain.
  **E.** None of the above.

_____ **73.** A potential complication for patients suffering from agricultural injuries is
  **A.** extended response and transport times.
  **B.** extended time to detection of the accident.
  **C.** possible contamination with manure.
  **D.** possible contamination by farm chemicals.
  **E.** all of the above.

# Chapter 8: Responding to Terrorist Acts

_____ **74.** Conventional explosives are the most common weapon terrorists use.
  **A.** True
  **B.** False

_____ **75.** In general, after a terrorist attack, the scene is safe to enter, as the damage of contamination and disease transmission passes very quickly.
  **A.** True
  **B.** False

_____ **76.** Which types of injuries associated with a nuclear ignition are the most lethal?
  **A.** Penetrating trauma          **D.** Burn injuries
  **B.** Blunt trauma                **E.** All of the above
  **C.** Compressional injuries

_____ **77.** After a nuclear detonation, the immediate area is likely to be radiation free for
  **A.** the first 2 minutes.        **D.** the first hour.
  **B.** 2 miles or more.            **E.** none of the above.
  **C.** 4 miles.

_____ **78.** The aspect of a nuclear blast that will affect persons the greatest distance from the epicenter is
  **A.** initial radiation.          **D.** structural collapse.
  **B.** fallout.                     **E.** electromagnetic pulse.
  **C.** burns.

_____ **79.** During a response to a suspected nuclear incident, you will likely wear a dosimeter, a pen-like device used to record your total radiation exposure.
  **A.** True
  **B.** False

____ 80. The radiation injury patient who has been properly decontaminated presents no danger to care providers.
- A. True
- B. False

____ 81. Generally, the patients who present with the earliest and most severe signs of radiation exposure are the least severely affected.
- A. True
- B. False

____ 82. Which of the following locations is a likely place for a chemical weapon attack?
- A. Subway
- B. Large building
- C. Shopping mall
- D. Convention center
- E. All of the above

____ 83. Which of the following chemical agents is classified as a nerve agent?
- A. Lewisite
- B. Ricin
- C. VX
- D. Mustard
- E. All of the above

____ 84. The first medication administered to a victim of nerve agent release is
- A. nitroglycerin.
- B. amyl nitrate.
- C. atropine.
- D. pralidoxime chloride.
- E. none of the above.

____ 85. The smell of newly mown grass is often associated with which chemical agent?
- A. Mace
- B. Hydrogen sulfide
- C. Botulinum
- D. Phosgene
- E. None of the above

____ 86. Which of the following biological agents is considered eradicated as a naturally occurring disease?
- A. Ebola
- B. Tularemia
- C. Anthrax
- D. Smallpox
- E. Q fever

____ 87. The first sign that a biological weapon attack has taken place may be numerous patients displaying flulike symptoms out of season.
- A. True
- B. False

____ 88. EMS and emergency department workers are at special risk for disease induced by biological agents when an attack occurs.
- A. True
- B. False

____ 89. A biological agent release is likely to be recognized early as a cloud of gas or particles or by the presentation of immediate signs and symptoms.
- A. True
- B. False

____ 90. The most effective action against biological agents is the use of personal protective equipment (Standard Precautions).
- A. True
- B. False

©2013 Pearson Education, Inc.
*Paramedic Care: Principles & Practice, Vol. 7, 4th Ed.*

_____ 91. Which of the following is a reason to be concerned about safety at the scene of a potential terrorist attack?
   A. Chemical agents may linger.
   B. Radiation danger may remain.
   C. Terrorists may set off secondary explosions.
   D. Biological agents carry risk of disease transmission.
   E. All of the above.

_____ 92. Your first role in responding to a possible act of terrorism is to ensure your own safety and that of your patient, other rescuers, and the public.
   A. True
   B. False

_____ 93. Once a WMD incident is identified, begin preparing for the casualties. Often this will entail instituting the Incident Command System and establishing the
   A. extrication sector.
   B. triage and treatment sectors.
   C. transport sector.
   D. decontamination sector.
   E. all of the above.

# WORKBOOK ANSWER KEY

*Note: Throughout the Answer Key, textbook page references are shown in italics.*

## Chapter 1: Ground Ambulance Operations

### CONTENT SELF-EVALUATION

#### MULTIPLE CHOICE

| | | | | | | | | |
|---|---|---|---|---|---|---|---|---|
| 1. | A | *p. 2* | 8. | D | *p. 5* | 15. | A | *p. 9* |
| 2. | A | *p. 3* | 9. | C | *p. 6* | 16. | C | *p. 9* |
| 3. | C | *p. 3* | 10. | B | *p. 6* | 17. | E | *p. 9* |
| 4. | E | *p. 3* | 11. | B | *p. 6* | 18. | B | *p. 10* |
| 5. | C | *p. 3* | 12. | B | *p. 7* | 19. | B | *p. 10* |
| 6. | B | *p. 4* | 13. | D | *p. 8* | 20. | B | *p. 10* |
| 7. | C | *p. 4* | 14. | B | *p. 8* | 21. | B | *p. 10* |

#### MATCHING

| | | | | | | | | |
|---|---|---|---|---|---|---|---|---|
| 22. | D | *p. 5* | 26. | E | *p. 5* | 30. | H | *p. 6* |
| 23. | F | *p. 2* | 27. | B | *p. 5* | 31. | G | *p. 6* |
| 24. | I | *p. 2* | 28. | C | *p. 6* | | | |
| 25. | A | *p. 5* | 29. | J | *p. 6* | | | |

### SPECIAL PROJECT

Answers will depend upon state motor vehicle laws and the standard operating procedures (SOPs) in the area where you will be serving as a paramedic.

## Chapter 2: Air Medical Operations

### CONTENT SELF-EVALUATION

#### MULTIPLE CHOICE

| | | | | | | | | |
|---|---|---|---|---|---|---|---|---|
| 1. | E | *p. 15* | 8. | E | *p. 21* | 15. | C | *p. 27* |
| 2. | B | *p. 17* | 9. | C | *p. 17* | 16. | C | *p. 28* |
| 3. | E | *p. 17* | 10. | D | *p. 26* | 17. | D | *p. 28* |
| 4. | A | *p. 17* | 11. | D | *p. 26* | 18. | B | *p. 28* |
| 5. | B | *p. 19* | 12. | A | *p. 26* | 19. | B | *p. 28* |
| 6. | C | *p. 20* | 13. | E | *p. 27* | 20. | E | *p. 29* |
| 7. | A | *p. 21* | 14. | B | *p. 27* | | | |

#### MATCHING

| | | |
|---|---|---|
| 21. | C | *p. 16* |
| 22. | D | *p. 17* |
| 23. | A | *p. 17* |
| 24. | E | *p. 19* |
| 25. | B | *p. 20* |

### SPECIAL PROJECT

The answers will vary with the state, region, or locale where you live.

## Chapter 3: Multiple-Casualty Incidents and Incident Management

### CONTENT SELF-EVALUATION

#### MULTIPLE CHOICE

| | | | | | | | | |
|---|---|---|---|---|---|---|---|---|
| 1. | C | *p. 37* | 11. | D | *p. 42* | 21. | A | *p. 48* |
| 2. | B | *p. 37* | 12. | A | *p. 42* | 22. | E | *p. 51* |
| 3. | A | *p. 38* | 13. | A | *p. 43* | 23. | A | *p. 51* |
| 4. | C | *p. 39* | 14. | C | *p. 44* | 24. | C | *p. 48* |
| 5. | A | *p. 40* | 15. | A | *p. 44* | 25. | E | *p. 54* |
| 6. | A | *p. 40* | 16. | D | *p. 45* | 26. | B | *p. 55* |
| 7. | A | *p. 41* | 17. | D | *p. 45* | 27. | A | *p. 56* |
| 8. | A | *p. 41* | 18. | B | *p. 46* | 28. | A | *p. 57* |
| 9. | A | *p. 41* | 19. | A | *p. 47* | 29. | A | *p. 58* |
| 10. | E | *p. 42* | 20. | D | *p. 47* | 30. | E | *p. 58* |

#### MATCHING

| | | | | | | | | |
|---|---|---|---|---|---|---|---|---|
| 31. | D | *p. 39* | 35. | A | *p. 44* | 39. | F | *p. 38* |
| 32. | J | *p. 44* | 36. | B | *p. 41* | 40. | E | *p. 41* |
| 33. | I | *p. 44* | 37. | G | *p. 43* | | | |
| 34. | H | *p. 40* | 38. | C | *p. 45* | | | |

### SHORT ANSWER

41. Multiple-/mass-casualty incident
42. Command, finance, logistics, operations, planning
43. Incident Management System
44. Simple Triage and Rapid Transport
45. Sort, assess, lifesaving interventions, treatment/transport

### SPECIAL PROJECT

Your plan should reflect local standard operating procedures (SOPs) and any other guidelines that affect your state or region. Ask a classmate or member of the EMS unit where you work to review your plan to ensure that you have thought of all contingencies. Then go one step further—test your plan in a tabletop drill, working out any wrinkles.

## Chapter 4: Rescue Awareness and Operations

### CONTENT SELF-EVALUATION

#### MULTIPLE CHOICE

| | | | | | | | | |
|---|---|---|---|---|---|---|---|---|
| 1. | E | *p. 63* | 8. | D | *p. 72* | 15. | B | *p. 82* |
| 2. | B | *p. 64* | 9. | E | *p. 72* | 16. | B | *p. 83* |
| 3. | D | *p. 66* | 10. | C | *p. 72* | 17. | D | *p. 84* |
| 4. | C | *p. 68* | 11. | E | *p. 75* | 18. | B | *p. 84* |
| 5. | C | *p. 68* | 12. | A | *p. 76* | 19. | A | *p. 86* |
| 6. | C | *p. 69* | 13. | C | *p. 76* | 20. | C | *p. 88* |
| 7. | A | *p. 72* | 14. | B | *p. 80* | | | |

MATCHING

**21.** H *p. 70*    **25.** J *p. 82*    **29.** G *p. 82*
**22.** C *p. 69*    **26.** I *p. 87*    **30.** B *p. 75*
**23.** F *p. 72*    **27.** D *p. 83*
**24.** A *p. 72*    **28.** E *p. 74*

## SPECIAL PROJECT

The answers will depend upon the resources in your area or region. As suggested in this chapter, you might try to participate in preplanning exercises in which some of these specialized agencies are involved.

# Chapter 5: Hazardous Materials

## CONTENT SELF-EVALUATION

### MULTIPLE CHOICE

**1.** E *p. 94*    **10.** B *p. 99*    **19.** A *p. 106*
**2.** A *p. 94*    **11.** B *p. 101*    **20.** D *p. 107*
**3.** B *p. 94*    **12.** B *p. 103*    **21.** D *p. 107*
**4.** C *p. 94*    **13.** D *p. 103*    **22.** D *p. 108*
**5.** D *p. 95*    **14.** A *p. 103*    **23.** C *p. 108*
**6.** A *p. 96*    **15.** A *p. 104*    **24.** A *p. 109*
**7.** B *p. 98*    **16.** A *p. 105*    **25.** E *p. 110*
**8.** C *p. 98*    **17.** A *p. 105*
**9.** B *p. 99*    **18.** A *p. 106*

### MATCHING

**26.** D *p. 93*    **30.** J *p. 101*    **34.** A *p. 101*
**27.** H *p. 96*    **31.** B *p. 101*    **35.** F *p. 101*
**28.** I *p. 99*    **32.** G *p. 101*
**29.** C *p. 99*    **33.** E *p. 101*

## SPECIAL PROJECT

Part I should accurately summarize the regulations and standards as they apply to you or your agency.
Part II will depend upon the chemicals selected.

# Chapter 6: Crime Scene Awareness

## CONTENT SELF-EVALUATION

### MULTIPLE CHOICE

**1.** B *p. 113*    **10.** A *p. 116*    **19.** C *p. 119*
**2.** B *p. 114*    **11.** B *p. 117*    **20.** B *p. 120*
**3.** B *p. 114*    **12.** E *p. 117*    **21.** B *p. 121*
**4.** C *p. 114*    **13.** E *p. 117*    **22.** E *p. 122*
**5.** A *p. 115*    **14.** B *p. 117*    **23.** A *p. 123*
**6.** E *p. 115*    **15.** A *p. 117*    **24.** A *p. 123*
**7.** A *p. 115*    **16.** B *p. 118*    **25.** E *p. 124*
**8.** B *p. 116*    **17.** E *p. 118*
**9.** C *p. 116*    **18.** B *p. 119*

### MATCHING

**26.** J *p. 117*    **30.** I *p. 122*    **34.** G *p. 123*
**27.** D *p. 121*    **31.** B *p. 124*    **35.** F *p. 122*
**28.** C *p. 120*    **32.** A *p. 114*
**29.** E *p. 121*    **33.** H *p. 120*

## SHORT ANSWER

### Part A

*pp. 123–124*

**36.** Avoid mixing samples of blood whenever possible.
**37.** Avoid tracking blood on your shoes.
**38.** If you must cut bloody clothing from a victim, place each piece in a separate brown paper bag. If the garment is wet, gently roll it in the paper bag to layer it. Place the entire contents in a second paper bag and then in a plastic bag for body fluid protection.
**39.** Do not throw clothes stained with blood or other body fluids in a single pile or in a puddle of blood.
**40.** Do not clean up or smudge blood splatters left at a scene.
**41.** If you leave behind blood from a venipuncture, notify the police.
**42.** Because blood can be a biohazard, ask police whether the scene should be secured for evidence collection.

### Part B

*pp. 123–124*

**43.** Prints (fingerprints, footprints, tire prints)
**44.** Particulate evidence
**45.** On-scene observations

## SPECIAL PROJECT

Items in the list will vary with the objects in your residence. Compare your list with the "weapons" identified by your classmates.

# Chapter 7: Rural EMS

## CONTENT SELF-EVALUATION

### MULTIPLE CHOICE

**1.** D *p. 128*    **5.** C *p. 130*    **9.** E *p. 134*
**2.** E *p. 128*    **6.** A *p. 131*    **10.** A *p. 138*
**3.** A *p. 129*    **7.** D *p. 133*
**4.** B *p. 129*    **8.** B *p. 133*

### MATCHING

**11.** E *p. 129*    **15.** A *p. 133*    **19.** J *p. 133*
**12.** G *p. 131*    **16.** I *p. 133*    **20.** H *p. 129*
**13.** B *p. 133*    **17.** C *p. 133*
**14.** D *p. 133*    **18.** F *p. 134*

## SHORT ANSWER

**21.** Distance and time
**22.** Communication difficulties
**23.** Enrollment shortages
**24.** Inadequate opportunities for training and practice
**25.** Inadequate medical support

©2013 Pearson Education, Inc.
*Paramedic Care: Principles & Practice, Vol. 7, 4th Ed.*

## SPECIAL PROJECT

*Answers will vary. You should look for the following:*

- Rural and Frontier Medical Services Toward the Year 2000 (paper on the future of rural EMS)
- Rural Emergency Medical Services Initiative (one state's program to assist with rural EMS)
- Pediatric Emergency Medicine in the Rural EMS System (paper on rural EMS)
- Rural Medics (a homepage for rural EMS providers)

## Chapter 8: Responding to Terrorist Acts

### CONTENT SELF-EVALUATION

#### MULTIPLE CHOICE

| | | | | | | | | |
|---|---|---|---|---|---|---|---|---|
| 1. | A | *p. 143* | 8. | C | *p. 145* | 15. | D | *p. 147* |
| 2. | E | *p. 143* | 9. | A | *p. 145* | 16. | E | *p. 148* |
| 3. | D | *p. 143* | 10. | E | *p. 145* | 17. | D | *p. 149* |
| 4. | B | *p. 143* | 11. | E | *p. 146* | 18. | E | *p. 151* |
| 5. | B | *p. 144* | 12. | A | *p. 146* | 19. | A | *p. 149* |
| 6. | E | *p. 145* | 13. | B | *p. 146* | 20. | A | *p. 150* |
| 7. | D | *p. 145* | 14. | C | *p. 146* | | | |

#### SPECIAL PROJECT

Part I : Salivation, lacrimation, urination, diarrhea, gastrointestinal distress, emesis

Part II: Atropine, pralidozime

## Operations: Content Review

### CONTENT SELF-EVALUATION

#### CHAPTER 1: GROUND AMBULANCE OPERATIONS

| | | | | | | | | |
|---|---|---|---|---|---|---|---|---|
| 1. | E | *p. 4* | 4. | B | *p. 6* | 7. | B | *p. 9* |
| 2. | B | *p. 5* | 5. | D | *p. 7* | 8. | A | *p. 10* |
| 3. | C | *p. 5* | 6. | B | *p. 9* | | | |

#### CHAPTER 2: AIR MEDICAL OPERATIONS

| | | | | | | | | |
|---|---|---|---|---|---|---|---|---|
| 9. | D | *p. 17* | 13. | B | *p. 25* | 17. | B | *p. 29* |
| 10. | B | *p. 19* | 14. | B | *p. 26* | 18. | D | *p. 30* |
| 11. | D | *p. 17* | 15. | A | *p. 27* | | | |
| 12. | D | *p. 21* | 16. | D | *p. 27* | | | |

#### CHAPTER 3: MULTIPLE-CASUALTY INCIDENTS AND INCIDENT MANAGEMENT

| | | | | | | | | |
|---|---|---|---|---|---|---|---|---|
| 19. | A | *p. 37* | 23. | A | *p. 41* | 27. | C | *p. 51* |
| 20. | B | *p. 38* | 24. | C | *p. 44* | 28. | D | *p. 55* |
| 21. | C | *p. 39* | 25. | D | *p. 44* | | | |
| 22. | D | *p. 40* | 26. | D | *p. 46* | | | |

#### CHAPTER 4: RESCUE AWARENESS AND OPERATIONS

| | | | | | | | | |
|---|---|---|---|---|---|---|---|---|
| 29. | D | *p. 63* | 34. | E | *p. 69* | 39. | E | *p. 76* |
| 30. | A | *p. 66* | 35. | D | *p. 72* | 40. | A | *p. 80* |
| 31. | E | *p. 67* | 36. | E | *p. 72* | 41. | B | *p. 84* |
| 32. | E | *p. 67* | 37. | B | *p. 72* | 42. | C | *p. 85* |
| 33. | A | *p. 67* | 38. | C | *p. 76* | 43. | E | *p. 87* |

#### CHAPTER 5: HAZARDOUS MATERIALS

| | | | | | | | | |
|---|---|---|---|---|---|---|---|---|
| 44. | A | *p. 94* | 48. | A | *p. 99* | 52. | B | *p. 104* |
| 45. | E | *p. 95* | 49. | A | *p. 101* | 53. | D | *p. 109* |
| 46. | C | *p. 96* | 50. | B | *p. 101* | | | |
| 47. | B | *p. 96* | 51. | A | *p. 102* | | | |

#### CHAPTER 6: CRIME SCENE AWARENESS

| | | | | | | | | |
|---|---|---|---|---|---|---|---|---|
| 54. | C | *p. 113* | 58. | B | *p. 118* | 62. | B | *p. 123* |
| 55. | E | *p. 113* | 59. | D | *p. 119* | 63. | E | *p. 123* |
| 56. | A | *p. 116* | 60. | D | *p. 122* | | | |
| 57. | D | *p. 117* | 61. | B | *p. 123* | | | |

#### CHAPTER 7: RURAL EMS

| | | | | | | | | |
|---|---|---|---|---|---|---|---|---|
| 64. | A | *p. 128* | 68. | E | *p. 131* | 72. | D | *p. 138* |
| 65. | C | *p. 129* | 69. | E | *p. 131* | 73. | E | *p. 136* |
| 66. | B | *p. 130* | 70. | E | *p. 132* | | | |
| 67. | D | *p. 131* | 71. | D | *p. 133* | | | |

#### CHAPTER 8: RESPONDING TO TERRORIST ACTS

| | | | | | | | | |
|---|---|---|---|---|---|---|---|---|
| 74. | A | *p. 143* | 81. | B | *p. 145* | 88. | A | *p. 151* |
| 75. | B | *p. 144* | 82. | E | *p. 146* | 89. | B | *p. 151* |
| 76. | D | *p. 145* | 83. | C | *p. 146* | 90. | A | *p. 150* |
| 77. | D | *p. 145* | 84. | C | *p. 146* | 91. | E | *p. 151* |
| 78. | B | *p. 145* | 85. | D | *p. 148* | 92. | A | *p. 152* |
| 79. | A | *p. 145* | 86. | D | *p. 150* | 93. | E | *p. 152* |
| 80. | A | *p. 145* | 87. | A | *p. 151* | | | |